POCKET GUIDE TO
Fetal Monitoring and Assessment

POCKET GUIDE TO

Fetal Monitoring and Assessment

Susan Martin Tucker, MSN, RN, PHN, CNAA

Healthcare Consultant
Quality Management and Perinatal Systems
Roseville, California

Fourth Edition

with 167 illustrations

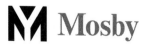

Mosby

An Imprint of Elsevier Science

St. Louis   London   Philadelphia   Sydney   Toronto

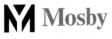

Mosby

An Imprint of Elsevier Science

Vice President, Nursing Editorial
Director: Sally Schrefer
Senior Editor: Michael S. Ledbetter
Editorial Assistant: Laura Selkirk
Project Manager: John Rogers
Senior Production Editor: Beth Hayes
Designer: Kathi Gosche
Cover photograph courtesy Lennart
Nilsson/Albert Bonniers Förlag AB,
A CHILD IS BORN, Dell Publishing
Company

Fourth Edition
Copyright © 2000
by Mosby, Inc.
Previous editions copyrighted
1988, 1992, 1996

NOTICE

Pharmacology is an ever-changing field. Standard safety precautions must be followed, but as new research and clinical experience broaden our knowledge, changes in treatment and drug therapy may become necessary or appropriate. Readers are advised to check the most current product information provided by the manufacturer of each drug to be administered to verify the recommended dose, the method and duration of administration, and contraindications. It is the responsibility of the appropriately licensed health care provider, relying on experience and knowledge of the patient, to determine dosages and the best treatment for each individual patient. Neither the publisher nor the editor assume any liability for any injury and/or damage to persons or property arising from this publication.

The Publisher

Mosby, Inc.
An Imprint of Elsevier Science
11830 Westline Industrial Drive
St. Louis, Missouri 63146
Printed in the United States of America

ISBN 0-323-00884-4
02 03 04 CL/FF 9 8 7 6 5 4 3

Contributors

MEREDITH FRESQUEZ, BSN, RNC, RDMS
Perinatal Study Coordinator/Perinatal Sonographer
Professional Education Center
Harbor/UCLA Medical Center
Los Angeles, California

DODI GAUTHIER, MEd, RNC
Perinatal Outreach Coordinator
Maternal Transport Coordinator
Santa Barbara Cottage Hospital
Santa Barbara, California

EVELYN HOM, MS, RN, CNS
Perinatal Clinical Nurse Specialist
San Francisco General Hospital Medical Center
San Francisco, California

JUDITH JOHNSON, BSN, RNC
Nurse Clinician
The Birth Center
Saint Joseph's Hospital
Marshfield, Wisconsin

TERRI NEGRON, MN, RN, FNP
Perinatal Clinical Coordinator
Crawford Long Hospital of Emory Healthcare
Atlanta, Georgia

CATHERINE ROMMAL, BS, RNC, FASHRM
Manager of Educational Services and Product
    Development
Farmers Insurance
Professional Liability Division
Malibu, California

Consultants

LINDA FOLEY, RN, MSN, PhD
Associate Chair of Curriculum
Nebraska Methodist College
Omaha, Nebraska

RHONDA HARWELL, MSN, RNC
Valley Perinatal Medical Group
Tarzana, California

MARTINA LETKO PORTER, MS, RNC, MBA
Market Development Manager for The Americas
Nellcor Perinatal Business
Mallinckrodt, Inc.
Pleasanton, California

KATHLEEN RUSSELL, RNC, MSN
Professor
Front Range Community College
Westminster, Colorado

BOBBIE TINNION, BA(Hons), RM, RN, ADM, MTD
Lecturer
School of Nursing and Midwifery
University of East Anglia
Norwich, Norfolk, England

DENA TOWNER, MD
Assistant Professor
Division of Maternal-Fetal Medicine
Perinatal Genetics
Director of Perinatal Diagnosis
Obstetrics and Gynecology
University of California Davis Medical Center
Davis, California

BARBARA F. WELLER, MSc, RGN, RSCN, RNT
Professional Officer
Neonatal Nurses Association
United Kingdom

Acknowledgments

AGILENT TECHNOLOGIES
Böblingen, Germany

SABARATNAM ARULKUMARAN, PhD, FRCS (Ed), FRCOG
Professor
Department of Obstetrics and Gynaecology
The University of Nottingham,
United Kingdom

ASSOCIATION OF WOMEN'S HEALTH, OBSTETRIC AND NEONATAL NURSES
Washington, D.C.

GERARD J. COLENBRANDER, MSEE
Department of Clinical Physics and Informatics
University Hospital, Vrije Universiteit
Amsterdam, The Netherlands

JUDITH ANN DOWD, MLS
Medical Department Administrator
Health Sciences Library
Kaiser Permanente Medical Center
Los Angeles, California

JIM FIORA STUDIOS
Wallingford, Connecticut

GE MARQUETTE MEDICAL SYSTEMS
Milwaukee, Wisconsin

HILL-ROM COMPANY, INC.
Batesville, Indiana

KAREN LEE, RDMS
Ultrasonographer
Mercy Perinatal Diagnostic Center
Mercy Healthcare
Sacramento, California

DENISE R. LUCAS, MSN, RNC
Staff Nurse
Labor and Delivery
Tri-Health Bethesda North Hospital
Cincinnati, Ohio

MALLINCKRODT, INC.
Nellcor Perinatal Business
Pleasanton, California

MEDICAL AND SCIENTIFIC ILLUSTRATIONS
Crozet, Virginia

LENNART NORDSTRÖM, MD
Associate Professor
South Hospital, Karolinska Institute
Stockholm, Sweden

ANN SHIELDS, BSN, RN
Labor and Delivery
Landstuhl Regional Medical Center
Landstuhl, Germany

CAROL THOROGOOD, MSN, RN
Coordinator of Midwifery Studies
Curtin University
Perth, Western Australia

HERMAN P. VAN GEIJN, MD, PhD
Professor in Obstetrics and Gynecology
Chairman of Obstetrics
Department of Obstetrics and Gynecology
Academic Hospital, Vrije Universiteit
Amsterdam, The Netherlands

Preface

Welcome to *the* most practical and portable book on fetal monitoring and assessment. The fourth edition of *Fetal Monitoring and Assessment* focuses on care of the fetal/maternal patient during the antepartum and intrapartum periods. The book has been thoroughly revised and updated to provide readily accessible, state-of-the-art information and to promote evidence-based practice of the healthcare professionals and students who care for these patients within our global community.

This book presents the theory and application of concepts of antepartum and intrapartum fetal monitoring and assessment. Principles of auscultation and use of electronic fetal monitoring/cardiotocography equipment and technology are described. Fetal heart rate patterns with analysis of monitor tracings are provided with protocols for interventions. Antepartum biophysical and biochemical monitoring techniques are presented. Patient care management protocols are provided for the care of the patient in labor, management of nonreassuring fetal heart rate patterns, initiation of labor, dysfunctional labor patterns, and preterm labor. Perinatal information systems with fetal surveillance and archival capabilities are described in addition to maternal/fetal risk factors, risk management, documentation, competency, and educational guidelines. Some of the unique features of this book are, as follows:

- The content of this book features a logical and progressive sequence of information. Both advanced concepts and basic elements are provided to augment the information base for experienced clinicians and to assist those who are new to the subject matter.
- Procedures and protocols are written in a step-by-step format and include rationales.
- To promote standardized intrapartum pattern interpretation by clinicians and investigators in an objective and consistent manner, a clear set of definitions for fetal heart rate patterns by the National Institute of Child Health and Human Development are provided to contribute to evidence-based clinical management.
- Clear explanations of physiological processes are presented for identifiable fetal heart rate patterns, and pathophysiology is presented for nonreassuring FHR patterns.

- An outline format in many sections serves to make the content readily accessible to the user. This is enhanced with the use of multiple charts, tables, illustrations, and photographs.
- This portable pocket guide provides an easy-to-use single source of fetal monitoring information while providing instant access for information needed quickly.

Organization

Chapter 1 provides an overview of fetal monitoring and assessment.

Chapter 2 provides a detailed presentation of the physiological basis for monitoring and regulatory control of the fetal heart rate.

Chapter 3 presents the instrumentation and technology used in monitoring and expands the discussion of auscultation because its efficacy compares with electronic monitoring in low-risk patients. Procedures and rationales are provided for the application and use of equipment for external and internal monitoring. Troubleshooting of equipment, central display, surveillance, and information systems are discussed, as well as considerations for monitor purchase. NEW to this chapter is the use of equipment terminology and the monitor scaling system used for tracings at 1 cm/min paper speed that is used outside North America.

Chapter 4 presents uterine activity monitoring and discusses subjective (palpation) and objective quantification of the intensity of uterine contractions. NEW content has been added on monitoring the progression of labor and the use of Montevideo Units.

Chapters 5 and 6 present detailed information on baseline fetal heart rate and changes that are episodic or related to uterine activity. The content is designed so that the reader can identify and interpret the patterns and implement appropriate interventions for nonreassuring patterns. At the end of each chapter a table summarizes the identification and management of each specific pattern. NEW to these chapters are the use of the definitions of the National Institute of Child Health and Human Development and an expanded section on fetal arrhythmias.

Chapter 7 discusses and contrasts reassuring and nonreassuring patterns and lists rationales for interventions as part of the assessment and management of fetal status. A handy tool is provided for the rapid interpretation of tracings. A protocol is provided for amnioinfusion, and the intrapartum use of tocolytic drugs is discussed. Other methods of assessing fetal status are included with NEW information on fetal oxygen saturation monitoring, including equipment, sensor mechanics, interpretation of data, and patient management. This new modality may be the most significant improvement in assessing intrapartum fetal status in the presence of nonreassuring heart rate patterns by reliably identifying the fetus who is adequately oxygenated and the fetus who is not.

Chapter 8 presents the multiple methods of antepartum monitoring and includes the use of ultrasound, detailed information on the biophysical profile, and NEW ultrasonograms and other imaging methods. Amniocentesis, other sampling methods, and fetal movement are discussed. Procedures for Contraction Stress Testing and Non-Stress Testing are included, with a protocol for acoustic stimulation. NEW content is provided on the lack of efficacy of home uterine activity monitoring.

Chapter 9 discusses the standard of care for the monitored patient and focuses on documentation of the important elements of monitoring and delivering patient care.

Chapter 10 expands and explores risk management concepts, with a discussion of competency, accountability, and communication of pertinent information. Emphasis is placed on the importance of having an established chain of command/consultation to ensure quality outcomes and documentation archival-retrieval for medical-legal purposes.

- The appendixes are provided to augment the foregoing with information related to fetal monitoring and assessment of the antepartum and intrapartum patient.
- Maternal and fetal risk factors are listed in Appendix A to identify patients at risk. A procedure with illustrations for performing Leopold's maneuvers is provided in Appendix B.
- Appendix C presents protocols for cervical ripening with Prepidil and Cervidil and provides a NEW protocol for Cytotec. A plan of care for augmentation and induction of labor is included, with information on dysfunctional labor patterns and the Bishop scoring system.
- A protocol for care of the patient in preterm labor is provided in Appendix D, with current information on the most widely used tocolytics, including magnesium sulfate, nifedipine, and terbutaline.
- NEW guidelines for culturally sensitive obstetric care are included in Appendix E to support the provision of holistic

care. In addition basic standards of care for the patient in labor are provided that can be modified according to institutional policy and practice preference.

- Selected fetal heart rate patterns are provided in Appendix F at the 3 cm/min paper speed that is used in North America. These patterns can be used to reinforce pattern recognition by the experienced clinician or they can be used as a learning tool for those new to pattern recognition.
- Appendix G is NEW and presents Clinical Competencies and Education Guide: Antepartum and Intrapartum Fetal Heart Rate Monitoring from the Association of Women's Health, Obstetric and Neonatal Nurses to support educators, students, and nursing managers who are conjointly responsible for achieving and maintaining competency of those involved in fetal monitoring.
- To support our international colleagues in the global community a NEW Appendix H provides sample tracings and selected pattern interpretation at the 1 cm/min paper speed that is routinely used in many countries.
- A glossary of terms and abbreviations is provided, as well as a list of references and a bibliography of helpful resources and Web sites.

Fetal Monitoring and Assessment provides up-to-date information for professional nurses, nurse midwives, physicians, medical students, physician residents, technicians, and medical-legal and risk management professionals who have a theoretical background in obstetrics. It also provides essential concepts in a clear, concise, and easily understandable manner for those who are new to electronic monitoring/cardiotocography.

The author wishes to acknowledge the support of Larry Tucker and the roles of Karrie Tucker Stewart and Jill Tucker in making this book a meaningful endeavor as they were the impetus for its creation. Lauren, Kyle, and Erika Stewart are the impetus for its revision. It is hoped that those who use this book will be instrumental in optimizing the environment of the unborn and quality of life of the newborn.

Susan Martin Tucker

Contents

6 Periodic and Nonperiodic Changes, 96

Fetal Monitoring and Assessment

Overview of Fetal Monitoring

The Dilemma and the Direction

The infant mortality (death before age 1 year) rate for the United States in 1997 was 7.1 infant deaths per 1000 live-born infants. This is the lowest rate recorded and represents a decrease of 16.4% from the rate of 8.5 per 1000 for 1992. The leading cause of infant mortality, congenital anomalies, accounted for 22% of all infant deaths, whereas the second major cause of death was preterm/low-birthweight infants at 13.5%. Other leading causes of infant mortality in descending order were Sudden Infant Death Syndrome (SIDS); respiratory distress syndrome; problems related to complications of pregnancy; complications of placenta, cord, and membrane; accidents; perinatal infections; and intrauterine hypoxia and birth asphyxia.

The leading causes of infant death varied considerably by race and national origin. For black infants, disorders related to short gestation and unspecified low birthweight were the leading causes of infant death, with an infant mortality rate 4 times that for white infants. For Native American infants, rates for SIDS and accidents and adverse effects were each 3.2 times higher than those for white infants. For Hispanic, Asian, and Pacific Islander mothers, infant mortality rates from SIDS were lower than those for all white mothers.

Of interest is the dramatic increase in multiple births, the result in part to the increased use of fertility-enhancing therapies and to the shift in delayed childbearing. The number of live births in triplet, quadruplet, quintuplet, and other higher-order multiple gestations rose 19% in a single year between 1995 and 1996. Between 1980 and 1996 the rate of multiple births jumped from 37.0 per 100,000 births to 152.6 per 100,000 births (CDC, 1996, 1999).

In contrast to the dramatic rises, falls, and variations in the foregoing statistics, the incidence of cerebral palsy remains unchanged at about 2 cases per 1000 term infants over the past 25 years. It had been hoped that the incidence of cerebral palsy, and even mental

1

retardation, might be reduced by as much as 50% by the use of electronic fetal monitoring (also known as cardiotocography [CTG]). This information is important to the public, as well as the medical and legal professions, to promote understanding that cerebral palsy is not often caused by events during labor and that the cause in most cases remains unknown (MacDonald, 1996).

The original rationale for the introduction of fetal heart rate (FHR) monitoring was that it could serve as a screening test for asphyxia that is severe enough to cause neurological damage, including cerebral palsy. That is, it could allow the recognition of asphyxia at a sufficiently early stage so that timely obstetrical intervention would prevent asphyxia-induced brain damage (NICHD, 1997). However, a substantial body of evidence has disproved the hypothesis that electronic fetal monitoring would reduce long-term neurological impairment and cerebral palsy in electronically monitored newborns. Electronic monitoring has been no more effective in reducing the rates of low Apgar scores at birth and long-term neurological morbidity than intensive intrapartum auscultation (ACOG, 1995d). Of interest is that the use of electronic monitoring has been associated with an increase in the rate of cesarean deliveries. The debate about advantages and limitations continues with regard to perinatal morbidity and mortality, costs for health care, and litigation.

One of the major impediments to progress in the evaluation and investigation of FHR monitoring has been the lack of agreement in definitions and nomenclature of FHR patterns used in the literature. Although some common terms have been used, it has not been consistently possible to determine from most of the publications exactly what the authors used for definitions and quantification of the various patterns, including those patterns signifying jeopardy for the fetus (NICHD, 1997).

Because of the foregoing, the National Institutes of Health held a Research Planning Workshop to assess the research status of this clinically important area, with meetings held from May 1995 to November 1996. Several investigators with expertise in the field were brought together to propose a standardized and unambiguous described set of definitions that could be quantitated and to develop recommendations for investigative interpretation of intrapartum FHR tracings, in order to more meaningfully assess the predictive value of electronic monitoring in observational studies and clinical trials (NICHD, 1997). Those definitions are defined and so noted in this book. The participants of the workshop included representation from the United States, Canada, and the United Kingdom. It was understood that the definitions may change in the future based on the results of research findings. There was, however, relatively little variation in opinion regarding the definition of the normal FHR tracing and agreement that there is reasonably good evidence that such a tracing confers an extremely high predictability of a normally oxygenated fetus at the time it is obtained (NICHD, 1997). With the advent of fetal oxygen saturation (FSpO$_2$) monitoring, it is hoped that nonreassuring patterns can be further evaluated to determine the need for an expeditious delivery or the continuation of labor.

Historical Overview

Fetal heart tones were first heard and described in the seventeenth century. During the next 200 years physicians described fetal heart tones or sounds and uterine souffle in medical journals. Then in 1917 Dr. David Hillis, an obstetrician at the Chicago Lying-In Hospital, reported on the use of a head stethoscope, or fetoscope. The chief of staff at the same institution, Dr. J.B. DeLee, published a report regarding the use of a similar instrument to auscultate the fetal heart. Controversy developed when Dr. DeLee claimed to have had the idea before Dr. Hillis. The instrument that we know today as the fetoscope became known as the DeLee-Hillis stethoscope and has remained essentially unchanged in design and use.

The move to a higher level of technology was made in 1958 when Dr. Edward Hon of the Yale University School of Medicine published a report on continuous fetal electrocardiographic monitoring from the maternal abdomen. Dr. Caldeyro-Barcia of Uruguay and Dr. Hammacher of Germany reported their observations of FHR patterns associated with fetal distress in 1966 and 1967, respectively. In 1968 Dr. Ralph Benson et al reported results of the collaborative study commissioned by the National Institute of Neurologic Diseases and Blindness. Some 24,863 deliveries were evaluated, and it was demonstrated that there was no correlation between the FHR as determined using a fetoscope and neonatal condition, except in the most extreme circumstance. This was almost always fetal bradycardia auscultated before a terminal event. Ten years before Benson's report, Hon discovered the unreliability of counting FHR when he asked 15 obstetricians to count several rates from a tape recording of the fetal heart and found a wide divergence in their counting.

As investigators throughout the world made similar observations of FHR decelerations and fluctuations from the baseline, a confusing array of terminology developed. At an international conference on FHR monitoring in December, 1971 in New Jersey, and later in March, 1972 in Amsterdam, Drs. Hon and Caldeyro-Barcia and their colleagues developed standard nomenclature for FHR monitoring. However, agreement on paper speed and universal scales was not reached and remained somewhat variable during the 1970s.

Since the first generation of commercially available fetal monitors in the late 1960s, technological advances have improved the quality and accuracy of the tracing. There are several electronic FHR monitors on the market, with some variations in capabilities; however, the basic components are the same.

There has been widespread acceptance of electronic FHR monitoring since the 1970s, with the majority of patients monitored during all or part of their labors. The hope for this technology was that it could prevent all or most cases of cerebral palsy. In addition, it had been hoped that electronic fetal monitoring would be more sensitive and accurate than intermittent auscultation in detecting FHR patterns that indicate fetal compromise. However, neither of these premises has been realized.

The Present and the Future

The current status of electronic fetal monitoring, or cardiotocography, is described as being at an awkward stage, not having reached full maturity. However, within the global community there have been many benefits to the use of electronic fetal monitoring, including a further understanding of (patho-)physiology, knowledge of technical pitfalls and factors influencing FHR patterns, discipline in the classification and interpretation of FHR patterns, and availability of protocols as to how, when, and whom to monitor. In addition, other benefits include recognition that electronic fetal monitoring is an indirect parameter of fetal condition, only one parameter of fetal condition, and a screening technique. Its use has prompted the use of digital storage of FHR data and to quantified and objective FHR analyses, although there are continuing inconsistencies in some definitions throughout the world (van Geijn, 1998).

Currently available, single monitors have technology that integrates several fetal (heart rhythm, oxygen saturation, gross fetal body movements) and maternal (heart rhythm, electrocardiogram, oxygen saturation, blood pressure) variables. It is hoped that this integration will provide more opportunities for investigation, particularly in studies of the effects of changes in the maternal cardiovascular status on the condition of the fetus.

Physiological Basis for Monitoring

2

Electronic fetal monitoring provides a technique for assessment of uterofetoplacental physiology and the adequacy of fetal oxygenation. Characteristic fetal heart rate (FHR) patterns are demonstrated as the result of hypoxic and nonhypoxic stresses or stimulation to the uterofetoplacental unit. Therefore it is important to have a basic understanding of the factors involved in fetal oxygenation, including uteroplacental circulation and physiology of FHR regulation.

Placenta and Intervillous Space

The placenta serves as a liaison between the fetal and maternal circulations (Figure 2-1). Oxygenated blood is delivered to the fetus through the umbilical vein. Deoxygenated blood returns to the placental chorionic villi through the two umbilical arteries. The chorionic villi are tiny vascular branches of the placenta that extend into the intervillous space. Maternal blood spurts upward from the uterine spiral arterioles and spreads laterally at random into the intervillous space, completely surrounding and bathing the villi (Figure 2-2). Although maternal and fetal blood are separated by a thin membrane and do not mix, several mechanisms occur whereby substances are exchanged across the placental membrane.

Mechanisms Occurring Within Intervillous Space

The intervillous space acts as a depot for the exchange of oxygen and nutrients and provides for the elimination of waste products. Together with the chorionic villi it functions as a fetal lung, gastrointestinal tract, kidney, skin (for heat exchange), infection barrier, and moderator of acid-base balance (Table 2-1).

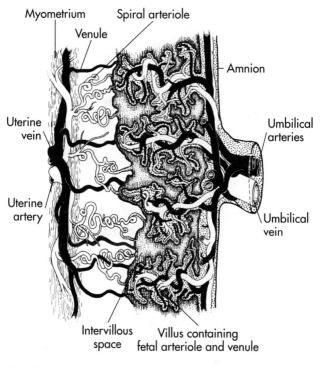

Figure 2-1
Schema of placenta.

At term some 700 to 800 ml of blood (10% to 15% of maternal cardiac output) perfuses the uterus each minute. Approximately 80% of this is within the intervillous space.

Exchange of Gases

Transport and transfer of respiratory gases are of critical importance to fetal survival. Oxygen and carbon dioxide exchange are complex processes that depend on many physiological and biochemical factors. These include intervillous space blood flow, diffusing capacity of the placenta, placental area and vascularity, membrane permeability and thickness, oxygen tension of uterine and umbilical blood vessels, hemoglobin affinity and hemoglobin concentration of maternal and fetal blood, and fetal umbilical cord

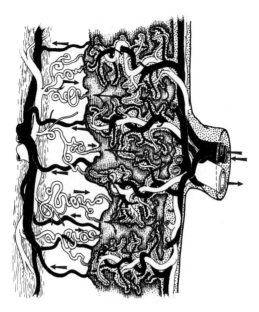

Figure 2-2
As maternal blood enters the intervillous space, it spurts upward from uterine spiral arterioles and spreads laterally at random.

blood flow. Intervillous space blood flow has already been described. Further description of the other factors follows.

Diffusing Capacity of Placenta

The diffusing capacity of the placenta regulates the rate of oxygen transfer by a concentration gradient and the rate of blood flow. Oxygen diffuses from the maternal blood, which has a higher partial pressure, to the fetal blood, which has a lower partial pressure. Maternal and fetal blood flow rates can be altered by decreases in maternal blood pressure (as occurs with supine hypotension and following conduction anesthesia such as spinal, caudal, or epidural anesthesia); maternal exercise, uterine hypertonus or polysystole, decreased placental surface area (abruptio placentae or infarcts); or by increases in blood pressure, such as occurs with preeclampsia or vasoconstricting drugs.

Table 2-1 Mechanisms occurring within the intervillous space

Mechanism	Description	Substances
Diffusion	Passage of substances from a region of higher concentration to one of lower concentration along a concentration gradient that is passive and requires no energy	Oxygen Carbon dioxide Small ions (sodium, chloride) Lipids Fat-soluble vitamins Many drugs
Facilitated diffusion	Substances pass on the basis of a concentration gradient; carrier molecule involved	Glucose Carbohydrates
Active transport	Passage of substances from one area to another against a concentration gradient; carrier molecules and energy are required	Amino acids Water-soluble vitamins Large ions (calcium, iron, iodine)
Bulk flow	Transfer of substances by a hydrostatic or osmotic gradient	Water Dissolved electrolytes
Pinocytosis	Transfer of minute, engulfed particles across a cell	Immune globulins Serum proteins
Breaks or leakage	Small breaks in the placental membrane allowing passage of substances	Maternal or fetal blood cells and plasma (potentially resulting in isoimmunization)

Placental Area

The larger and more vascular the placenta, the greater is the amount of substances that can be transferred between mother and fetus. Reduced placental area is associated with maternal hypertension, maternal diabetes, maternal vascular disease, fetal growth retardation, intrauterine infection, abruptio placentae, placenta previa, placental infarctions, and circumvallate placenta.

Oxygen Tension

Oxygen tension in maternal arterial blood is determined by adequate pulmonary function. Diminished function resulting from maternal disease process or hypoventilation will decrease arterial oxygen tension (arterial PO_2). Some of the conditions that decrease arterial oxygen tension include congestive heart failure, maternal congenital cardiac defects, cystic fibrosis, and chronic obstructive pulmonary diseases (asthma and emphysema). The addition of inspired oxygen can increase arterial oxygen tension (arterial PO_2).

Oxygen transfer from maternal to fetal hemoglobin is regulated by the oxygen tension of the umbilical blood vessels. Generally, oxygen tension of the umbilical vessels is much lower than that of the maternal vessels (Figure 2-3) (Helwig et al, 1996). Some factors that compensate for this low fetal oxygen tension follow:

1. Increased fetal cardiac output (three to four times that of the resting adult per kilogram of body weight) based on heart rate
2. Increased oxygen-carrying capacity caused by high hemoglobin values (as compared with adult blood)
3. Increased affinity of fetal blood for oxygen (as compared with adult blood) with a higher saturation of fetal hemoglobin at the same given PO_2 based on the fetal hemoglobin dissociation curve
4. Anatomical fetal shunts: ductus venosus, foramen ovale, and ductus arteriosis

Hemoglobin and Oxygen Affinity

Hemoglobin concentrations of maternal and fetal blood differ at term. Maternal hemoglobin is approximately 12 g/100 ml, in contrast with fetal hemoglobin, which is about 15 g/100 ml. Each gram of hemoglobin is capable of combining with 1.34 ml of oxygen. This increased oxygen-carrying capacity of fetal blood plus the high affinity of fetal blood for oxygen facilitate the transfer of oxygen from mother to fetus.

Oxygen saturation of hemoglobin is the relationship between the amount of oxygen that is carried on the hemoglobin and the amount of oxygen that can be carried. For example, a 90% saturation in the adult means that the hemoglobin is carrying 90% of its potential capacity. The amount of oxygen combined with hemoglobin depends on the partial pressure of oxygen (PaO_2) dissolved

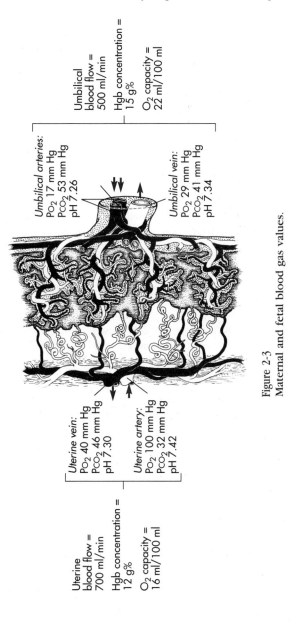

Umbilical
blood flow =
500 ml/min

Hgb concentration =
15 g%

O_2 capacity =
22 ml/100 ml

Umbilical arteries:
Po_2 17 mm Hg
Pco_2 53 mm Hg
pH 7.26

Umbilical vein:
Po_2 29 mm Hg
Pco_2 41 mm Hg
pH 7.34

Uterine vein:
Po_2 40 mm Hg
Pco_2 46 mm Hg
pH 7.30

Uterine artery:
Po_2 100 mm Hg
Pco_2 32 mm Hg
pH 7.42

Uterine
blood flow =
700 ml/min

Hgb concentration =
12 g%

O_2 capacity =
16 ml/100 ml

Figure 2-3
Maternal and fetal blood gas values.

in the arterial blood. The oxyhemoglobin saturation at different partial pressures vary, as demonstrated on a standard oxyhemoglobin dissociation curve. The curve is altered by changes in pH. This is known as the *Bohr effect*. The curve shifts to the right in the presence of an acidic pH and to the left in the presence of an alkaline pH. This changes the difference between the fetal and maternal curves and increases the gradient, which is beneficial for oxygen exchange.

The oxygen saturation of hemoglobin can be measured in the mother by *pulse oximetry (SpO_2)*. During the intrapartum period, *fetal oxygen saturation ($FSpO_2$)* can be measured to identify the fetal response to nonreassuring FHR patterns. Fetal oxygen saturation ($FSpO_2$) monitoring is discussed in Chapter 8.

Umbilical Blood Flow

The mechanical force of a uterine contraction impedes intervillous space blood flow, exerts pressure directly on the fetus, and can occlude blood flow in both directions through the umbilical cord. Rapid fetal asphyxia with hypoxemia and acidosis can occur with entrapment and compression of the cord between fetal parts and the uterine wall. Transient cord compression occurs in about 40% of all labors, and the fetus is usually able to compensate in the intervals between contractions. However, in some labors in which the cord prolapses or is short, knotted, wrapped around fetal body parts, or where oligohydramnios is present, uncorrectable and prolonged variable deceleration of the FHR occurs. This is an obstetrical emergency, usually requiring immediate operative intervention, because fetal asphyxiation and death can occur. Amnioinfusion, the instillation of normal saline or lactated Ringer's solution through an intrauterine catheter (a discussion of which can be found in Chapter 7), can act as a buffer between fetal parts and the uterine wall and can relieve variable decelerations caused by cord compression.

Uterine Blood Flow

The passage of critical substances across the placenta is determined by uterine blood flow. The flow of blood increases as pregnancy progresses so that by term about 700 ml of blood flows each minute. This volume is about 10% of the maternal cardiac output.

Uterine blood flow is determined by uterine arterial and venous pressures and uterine vascular resistance. Any impact on these three factors can alter uterine blood flow. Discussion of some of the causes of decreased uterine blood flow follows.

Maternal Position

A decrease in blood flow to the uterus can occur when the mother is in the dorsal recumbent position. The gravid uterus lies on the mother's vertebral column, exerting pressure on the great vessels, particularly the inferior vena cava. This pressure can compress the vessel, decreasing the volume of blood returning to the heart and producing a decrease in maternal cardiac output, hypotension, and a decrease in uterine blood flow. This mechanism is called *supine hypotension syndrome.*

Exercise

Fetal tachycardia that occurs after maternal exercise is thought to be caused by a transitory period of reduced fetal oxygenation. Although maternal exercise diverts blood to the muscle groups and away from the uterus, there is no evidence that exercise is harmful when there is normal uteroplacental function.

Uterine Contractions

Uterine contractions cause a decrease in the rate of perfusion of maternal blood through the intervillous space. Angiographic studies demonstrating this have shown impaired filling of the lobules with contrast medium during uterine contractions. In addition, fetal arterial blood oxygen tension decreases following the onset of each uterine contraction. The fetus, in most gestations, seems well able to compensate for these relatively minor stresses. However, in high-risk pregnancies in which the margin of fetal reserve is abnormally low, uterine contractions can cause some degree of hypoxia and commensurate decreases in the FHR, known as *late decelerations.* Recognition and treatment of late decelerations are described in Chapter 6.

To avoid compounding these stresses, it is important that the uterus relax adequately between contractions, that contractions not be excessively long, and that the tonus not rise. Intrauterine pressure between contractions—*resting tone (tonus)*—ranges from 5 to 15 mm Hg, with the average pressure between 8 and 12 mm Hg. During contractions intrauterine pressure ranges from 30 mm Hg to more than 80 mm Hg, with an intensity of 50 mm Hg to more than 100 mm Hg at the peak of the contraction. Angiographic studies show a cessation of maternal blood flow to the intervillous space with intrauterine pressures of 50 to 60 mm Hg during normal labor contractions.

It is thought that the fetus receives most of the oxygen and nutrients and eliminates most of the carbon dioxide (CO_2) between contractions while the uterus is at rest. Thus a healthy fetus with a normal placenta subjected to frequent contractions with inadequate uterine relaxation can become hypoxic and acidotic.

Uterine Hypertonus

Uterine hypertonus—excessively high intrauterine pressure—can also cause the fetus to experience stress. Uterine hypertonus may occur spontaneously in some patients, particularly in those with a very distended uterus, as a result of hydramnios, multiple gestation, or macrosomia. However, hypertonus is most frequently caused by uterine hyperstimulation with oxytocin. In some sensitive patients oxytocin produces hypertonus, characterized by high intrauterine pressure with absence of relaxation for a prolonged period. Abruptio placentae may also cause uterine hypertonus as a result of irritation of the myometrium from extravasated blood. In preeclampsia, uterine resting tone is elevated because of vasoconstriction, decreased uterine blood flow, and reduced placental surface area (Freeman, Garite, Nageotte, 1991). In addition, the following factors can interfere with placental perfusion and jeopardize the fetus:
1. Contractions lasting longer than 90 seconds
2. Periods of relaxation between contractions that are less than 30 seconds
3. Inadequate decrease in intrauterine pressure between contractions

Surface Area of Placenta

The potential for fetal hypoxia is increased with any reduction in the placental surface area. Abruptio placentae is a clear example of this. Reduced placental area exposes the fetus to uteroplacental insufficiency and is associated with infarcts (as in hypertensive or prolonged pregnancies), maternal vascular disease, maternal diabetes, intrauterine infection, placenta previa, or circumvallate placenta.

Conduction Anesthesia

Maternal hypotension caused by sympathetic blockade occurring with conduction anesthesia reduces blood flow in the intervillous space. Restoration of uterine blood flow is usually achieved by positional changes and expansion of maternal blood volume. Prehydration for women who are about to receive conduction anesthesia should be considered. Pressor agents, such as ephedrine, may also be required to restore maternal blood pressure.

Hypertension

Whether maternal hypertension is essential or pregnancy-induced, there is an increase in vascular resistance, resulting in a decrease in uterine blood flow.

Physiology of Fetal Heart Rate Regulation

The average FHR at term is 140 beats per minute (bpm). The normal range is 110 to 160 bpm. Earlier in gestation the FHR is slightly higher, with the average being approximately 160 bpm at 20 weeks' gestation (Freeman, Garite, Nageotte, 1991). The rate progressively decreases as the fetus reaches term.

Regulatory control of the FHR depends on multiple factors (Parer, 1997) as described in Table 2-2. The cerebral cortex, hypothalamus, and medulla oblongata are components of the central nervous system that influence FHR. The autonomic nervous system has two major divisions: the parasympathetic and the sympathetic nervous systems. The vagus nerve, which innervates the sinoatrial (SA) node and the atrioventricular (AV) node of the fetal heart, is the primary component of the parasympathetic nervous system. Stimulation of the vagus nerve produces cardiodeceleration. Stimulation of the sympathetic nervous system results in cardioacceleration. Baroreceptors are stretch receptors or pressoreceptors in the aortic arch and carotid sinus that respond to changes in blood pressure, effecting a change in FHR. Peripheral chemoreceptors located in carotid and aortic bodies can effect bradycardia, and central chemoreceptors located in the medulla oblongata can effect tachycardia. The schema of the relationship of these factors in regulating the FHR is depicted in Figure 2-4. Other factors that may influence the FHR are disturbances such as hyperthermia resulting in tachycardia and hypothermia resulting in bradycardia.

Table 2-2   Regulatory control of fetal heart rate (FHR)

Factors Regulating FHR	Location
Parasympathetic division of autonomic nerve system	Vagus (tenth cranial) nerve fibers supply sinoatrial (SA) and atrioventricular (AV) nodes
Sympathetic division of autonomic nervous system	Nerves widely distributed in myocardium
Baroceptors	Stretch receptors in aortic arch and carotid sinus at the junction of the internal and external carotid arteries
Chemoceptors	Peripheral—in carotid and aortic bodies

Central—in medulla oblongata |
| Central nervous system | Cerebral cortex

Hypothalamus

Medulla oblongata |
| Hormonal regulation | Adrenal medulla (Catecholamines) |

Action	Effect
Stimulation causes release of acetylcholine at myoneural synapse	Decreases FHR Maintains beat-to-beat variability
Stimulation causes release of norepinephrine at synapse	Increases FHR Increases strength of myocardial contraction Increases cardiac output
Responds to increase in blood pressure by stimulating stretch receptors to send impulses via vagus or glossopharyngeal nerve to midbrain, producing vagal response and slowing heart activity	Decreases FHR Decreases blood pressure Decreases cardiac output
Responds to a marked peripheral decrease in O_2 and increase in CO_2	Produces bradycardia, sometimes with increased variability
Central chemoceptors respond to decreases in O_2 tension and increases in CO_2 tension in blood and/or cerebrospinal fluid	Produces tachycardia and increase in blood pressure with decrease in variability
Responds to fetal movement	Increases reactivity and variability
Responds to fetal sleep	Decreases reactivity and variability
Regulates and coordinates autonomic activities (sympathetic and parasympathetic)	
Mediates cardiac and vasomotor reflex center by controlling heart action and blood vessel diameter	Maintains balance between cardioacceleration and cardiodeceleration; modulates variability
Releases epinephrine and norepinephrine with severe fetal hypoxia producing sympathetic response	Increases FHR Increases strength of myocardial contraction and blood pressure Increases cardiac output

Continued

Table 2-2   Regulatory control of fetal heart rate—cont'd

Factors Regulating FHR	Location
Hormonal regulation—cont'd	Adrenal cortex
	Pituitary neurohypophysis (vasopressin)
	Renal juxtaglomerular cells (renin-angiotensin II)
Blood volume/capillary fluid shift	Fluid shift between capillaries and interstitial spaces
Intraplacental pressures	Intervillous space
Frank-Starling mechanism	Based on stretching of myocardium by increased inflow of venous blood into right atrium

Action	Effect
Low fetal blood pressure stimulates release of aldosterone, decreases sodium output, increases water retention, which increases circulating blood volume	Maintains homeostasis of blood volume
Produces vasoconstriction of nonvital vascular beds in the asphyxiated fetus to increase blood pressure	Distributes blood flow to maintain FHR and variability; linked to sinusoidal pattern
Released when intraarterial volume low	Stimulates vasoconstriction to maintain blood pressure
Responds to elevated blood pressure by causing fluid to move out of capillaries and into interstitial spaces	Decreases blood volume and blood pressure
Responds to low blood pressure by causing fluid to move out of interstitial space into capillaries	Increases blood volume and blood pressure
Fluid shift between fetal and maternal blood is based on osmotic and blood pressure gradients; maternal blood pressure is about 100 mm Hg and fetal blood pressure about 55 mm Hg; therefore balance is probably maintained by some compensatory factor	Regulates blood volume and blood pressure
In the adult the myocardium is stretched by an increased inflow of blood, causing the heart to contract with greater force than before and pump out more blood; the adult then is able to increase cardiac output by increasing heart rate and stroke volume; this mechanism is not well-developed in the fetus	Cardiac output is dependent on heart rate in the fetus: ↓ FHR = ↓ cardiac output ↑ FHR = ↑ cardiac output

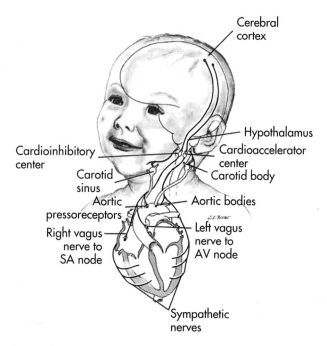

Figure 2-4
Schema of relation of control of FHR from central nervous system, parasympathetic and sympathetic divisions of autonomic nervous system, baroceptors, and chemoceptors.

In summary, regulatory control of the FHR, the quality and efficacy of uteroplacental circulation, umbilical blood flow, respiratory gas exchange, and fetal circulation are determining factors in the fetal response to labor. An understanding of these factors forms the basis of FHR and uterine activity monitoring.

Instrumentation for Fetal Heart Rate and Uterine Activity Monitoring

3

Overview

The goal of fetal heart rate (FHR) monitoring is to detect signs that warn of potential adverse events in order to provide intervention in a timely manner. The FHR can be monitored by intermittent auscultation or by electronic means with an external or internal device. This chapter presents a description of devices that can be used to monitor the FHR and includes information on uterine activity monitoring, central display terminals, and telemetry. In addition, factors to be considered before purchasing an electronic monitor are provided.

Auscultation of Fetal Heart Rate
Description

In addition to the use of the electronic fetal monitor, auscultation of the FHR may be performed with a stethoscope, DeLee-Hills fetoscope, Pinard stethoscope, or Doppler ultrasound device (Figure 3-1). Auscultation is a learned skill that improves with practice. Auscultation is *not* electronic fetal monitoring without a tracing. It is a *counting* technique in which an instrument (or a listening device) is used to count the number of fetal heart beats occurring in a prescribed amount of time and evaluated at a prescribed amount of time. The rate obtained is utilized, along with other assessment data, to guide management and care of the maternal-fetal dyad.

If a *stethoscope* is used, the end should be turned so that the domed side of the stethoscope, rather than the flat side, is open to

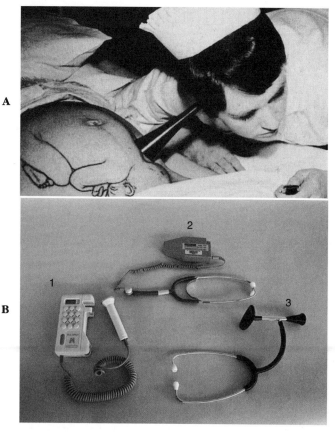

Figure 3-1

A, Auscultation of FHR with a Pinard stethoscope. Vertex left occipitoanterior. **B,** *1,* Ultrasound fetoscope. *2,* Ultrasound stethoscope. *3,* DeLee-Hillis fetoscope.

(A from Bennett VR, Brown LK, eds: *Myles textbook for midwives,* ed 13, London, Churchill Livingstone. B, Courtesy Michael S. Clement, MD, Mesa, Ariz.)

the connective tubing to the ear pieces. The domed side is then placed on the maternal abdomen. The *fetoscope* should be applied to the listener's head, because bone conduction amplifies the fetal heart sounds for counting. It is the ventricular fetal heart sounds that can be counted with the stethoscope and fetoscope. The *Doppler ultrasound* device transmits ultra–high-frequency sound waves to the moving interface of the fetal heart valves and deflects these back to the device, converting them into an electronic signal that can be counted.

Procedure	Rationale
1. Perform Leopold's maneuvers (see Appendix B) by palpating the maternal abdomen	1. To identify fetal presentation and position
2. Place the listening device over the area of maximum intensity, which is usually over the back of the fetus, and clarity of the fetal heart sounds	2. To obtain the clearest and loudest sound, which is easier to count
3. Count the maternal radial pulse	3. To differentiate it from the fetal rate
4. Palpate the abdomen for the absence of uterine activity	4. To be able to count FHR between contractions
5. Count the FHR for 30 or 60 seconds *between* contractions	5. To identify the baseline rate, which can only be assessed during the absence of uterine activity
6. Auscultate the FHR during a contraction, if possible, and for 30 seconds after the end of the contraction	6. To identify the FHR during the contraction and as a response to the contraction
7. When there are distinct discrepancies in FHR during or between listening periods, auscultate for a longer period during, after, and between contractions	7. To identify changes from the baseline that indicate the need for another mode of FHR monitoring

Frequency of Auscultation

Regardless of the method used to assess FHR, the standard practice is to evaluate and record the heart rate at specific intervals. The frequency of auscultation and documentation of the FHR is based on AAP/ACOG guidelines (1997) and AWHONN (1997) and SOGC standards (1995).

Stage of Labor	Low Risk	High Risk
Latent phase	q 30-60 minutes	q 30 minutes
Active phase	q 30 minutes	q 15 minutes
Second stage	q 15 minutes	q 5 minutes

Based on reviews of well-controlled studies, no differences in perinatal outcomes have been identified between intermittent auscultation and continuous electronic FHR monitoring (Vintzileos, 1995). This has been observed even in the presence of risk factors on admission or those appearing during the course of labor, when the FHR has been evaluated at the intervals described above (AAP/ ACOG, 1997). It is important to note that the studies did employ *a ratio of one nurse to one patient,* which should be employed if auscultation is used as the primary technique of FHR surveillance.

Auscultation of the FHR should occur *before* the administration of medications (including oxytocics and analgesics) and anesthetics, before periods of ambulation, and before artificial rupture of membranes. The FHR should be assessed immediately *following* rupture of membranes, changes in strength of uterine contraction (resting tone increase, sustained contraction, or tachysystole), vaginal examinations, changes in dosage of oxytocics, response to oxytocics, administration of medications (during peak action period), urinary catheterization, periods of ambulation, changes in dosage of anesthetic agents, and response to analgesics and anesthetics.

Many countries prefer the use of intermittent auscultation to continuous electronic fetal monitoring in patients without risk factors to promote patient mobility, provide less distraction, and provide a more natural birthing experience without the use of electrical devices. Reliance on the use of the electronic monitor is more prevalent in the United States, likely because of staffing patterns, staffing mix, and the increase of defensive practices in a litigious environment.

Documentation

Documentation of the FHR must be accompanied by other routine parameters that are assessed during labor, including uterine activity, maternal observations and assessment, and both maternal and fetal responses to interventions. It should be noted how long the heart rate was auscultated and whether this was before, during, and/or immediately after a uterine contraction. The rate, rhythm, and abrupt or gradual increases or decreases of the FHR during any part of this auscultated period should be described in relationship to the concurrent uterine activity. It is not appropriate to describe auscultated FHR using the descriptive terms associated with electronic fetal monitoring because the majority of the terms are visual descriptions of the patterns produced on the monitor tracing (e.g., *early*, *late*, and *variable decelerations*). However, terms that are numerically defined, such as *bradycardia* and *tachycardia*, can be used.

Interpretation of Auscultated Fetal Heart Rate
Reassuring fetal heart rate

- FHR in the normal heart rate range without wide fluctuations from the average rate (which is obtained between contractions), usually over a 10-minute period

Nonreassuring fetal heart rate

- A baseline FHR of <100 bpm or >160 bpm
- A decrease in the FHR of >30 bpm following a contraction
- Irregular cardiac rhythm

Management options of a nonreassuring fetal heart rate

- Increase frequency of auscultation
- Apply electronic fetal monitor to visualize pattern suspected or to assess baseline variability
- Intervene appropriately to promote uterine and umbilical blood flow, improve fetal oxygenation, and decrease uterine activity if excessive (AWHONN, 1997)
- Vibroacoustic stimulation with electronic monitoring to assess fetal response may be helpful
- Notify health care provider as appropriate

If nonreassuring FHR patterns persist after attempts to correct them have been made or if ancillary tests are not appropriate, then an expeditious delivery may be considered by the health care provider.

Advantages of auscultation of fetal heart rate

- Widely available and easy to use
- Noninvasive
- Inexpensive
- Comfortable for patient
- Provides freedom of patient movement
- Increases "hands-on" contact with patient

Limitations

- May require maternal supine position, which could predispose to supine hypotension syndrome
- Does not provide a permanent, documented record
- The counting of FHR is intermittent
- Cannot assess FHR variability or periodic changes
- Nonreassuring events may occur during unmonitored periods
- Does not allow for early detection of nonreassuring patterns

In summary, auscultatory FHR monitoring has been found to be effective if performed in a consistent manner by a nurse caring for a patient according to the prescribed frequency. Because of the time- and labor-intensive nature of this method of monitoring, it may not always be an option in a busy unit that has the capability of continuous electronic FHR monitoring.

Electronic Fetal Monitoring

There are two modes of electronic monitoring. The external, or indirect, mode employs the use of external transducers placed on the maternal abdomen to assess FHR and uterine activity. The internal, or direct, mode uses a spiral electrode to assess the FHR and variability and the intrauterine pressure catheter to assess uterine activity and intrauterine pressure (Figures 3-2, 3-3, and 3-4). In some countries the electronic fetal monitor is called a *cardiotocograph (CTG)*. A brief description contrasting the external and internal modes of monitoring with a more detailed explanation of application and use follows.

	External Mode (Indirect)	Internal Mode (Direct)
Fetal heart rate	Ultrasound (Doppler) transducer: High-frequency sound waves reflect mechanical action of fetal heart (easiest and most reliable external method to use during the antepartum and intrapartum periods)	Spiral electrode: Electrode converts fetal electrocardiogram (ECG) as obtained from presenting part to FHR via cardiotachometer by measuring consecutive fetal R wave intervals; this method can be used only when membranes are ruptured and the cervix is sufficiently dilated during the intrapartum period; electrode penetrates fetal presenting part 1.5 mm and must be securely attached to ensure a good signal
Uterine activity	Tocotransducer: This instrument monitors approximate frequency and duration of contractions by means of a pressure-sensing device applied to the abdomen; it can be used during antepartum and intrapartum periods	Intrauterine catheter: This instrument monitors frequency, duration, *intensity* of contractions, and resting tone; the catheter is compressed during contractions, placing pressure on a transducer tip or a strain gauge mechanism of a fluid-filled catheter and then converting the pressure into mm Hg on the uterine activity panel of the strip chart; it can be used only when membranes are ruptured and the cervix is sufficiently dilated during intrapartum period; these catheters are available with a second lumen that can be used for amnioinfusion

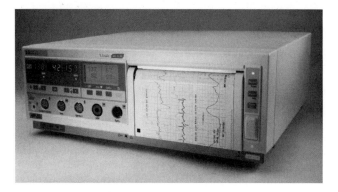

Figure 3-2
The Viridia 50 XM fetal/maternal monitor provides measurement of FHR, UA, gross fetal body movement, twin offset (to separate FHR tracings of twins for easier interpretation), and maternal parameters, including ECG, HR, noninvasive BP, and SpO_2. The Viridia 50 XMO monitors the foregoing with the addition of fetal oxygen saturation ($FSpO_2$).
(Courtesy Agilent Technologies, Böblingen, Germany.)

External Mode of Monitoring
Ultrasound transducer
Description

Ultrasonic high-frequency sound waves are transmitted by a transducer placed on the maternal abdomen. As the ultrasound strikes a moving interface—in this case the fetal heart ventricles—a signal is directed back to the transducer, activating a tachometer. The FHR is printed out on the upper part of the tracing or strip chart, and a simultaneous indicator light or audible beep on the monitor is activated with each heartbeat. This Doppler signal can be affected by changes in the position of the transducer or the fetus. Changes in the direction of the sound beam during uterine contractions may cause a loss of signal and make the resulting tracing uninterpretable. Because ultrasound reflects mechanical movement of the fetal heart, it cannot assess accurate short-term variability in the FHR. However, monitors with autocorrection capability very closely approximate accurate short-term variability. Autocorrelation works by matching each

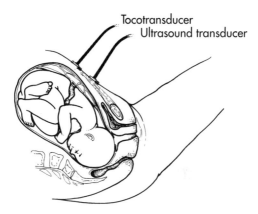

Tocotransducer
Ultrasound transducer

Figure 3-3
Placement of external transducers.

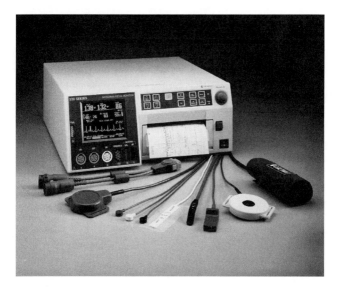

Figure 3-4
Corometrics Model 129 maternal/fetal monitor provides measurement of FHR, fetal oxygen saturation ($FSpO_2$), UA, and maternal parameters, including SpO_2, ECG, HR, and noninvasive BP. The audible and visual "Spectra Alert" option may be added to this monitor.
(Courtesy GE Marquette Medical Systems, Milwaukee, Wis. Photo by Jim Fiora.)

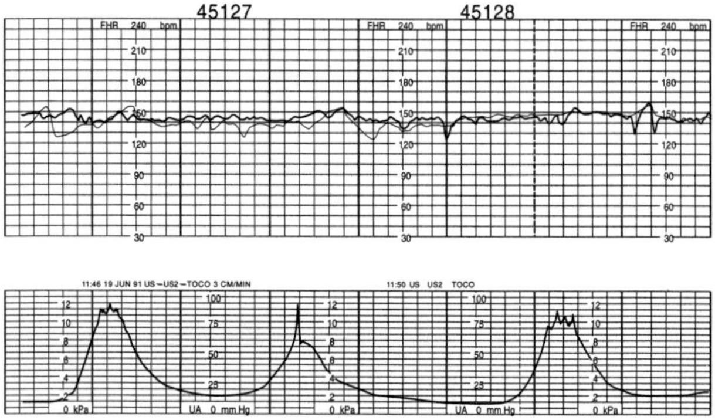

30   Chapter Three

Figure 3-5
Dual ultrasonic heart rate monitoring strip demonstrates the
simultaneous external monitoring of twins.
(Courtesy GE Marquette Medical Systems, Milwaukee, Wis.)

incoming waveform with the previous one and repetitively
analyzing small segments of those waveforms. Some monitors
have dual ultrasound channels for the simultaneous monitoring of
twins (Figure 3-5).

The ultrasound transducer can be used to monitor FHR during both the antepartum and intrapartum periods. Correct
placement of the ultrasound transducer depends on maternal
cooperation and operator skill, because the transducer usually
must be repositioned when the maternal position changes. Excessive fetal movement can cause erratic operation of the FHR
stylus. Very rapid changes in FHR, such as sudden variable
decelerations, may not be followed completely by the ultrasound
transducer.

The following information provides a step-by-step approach for
use of the ultrasound transducer.

Procedure	Rationale
1. Explain the procedure to the patient and her family	1. To allay anxiety

Procedure	Rationale
2. Gather necessary equipment: Fetal monitor, ultrasound transducer, and either toco-transducer or intrauterine catheter apparatuses (to assess uterine activity), ultrasonic coupling gel, and abdominal belt	2. To ensure that all equipment is readily accessible
3. Position the patient in a semilateral position of comfort	3. To avoid supine hypotension syndrome
4. Perform Leopold's maneuvers (see Appendix B)	4. To determine fetal position
5. Align and insert the ultrasound transducer plug into the appropriate monitor port labeled "cardio" or "US" for ultrasound	5. To provide connection without damaging connector pins, which could result in a faulty signal
6. Apply ultrasound coupling gel to the underside of the transducer placed on the maternal abdomen	6. To aid in the transmission of ultrasound waves
7. Place the transducer on the abdomen, preferably over the fetal back or below the level of the umbilicus in a full-term pregnancy of cephalic presentation or above the level of the umbilicus in a full-term pregnancy of breech presentation	7. To search for the clearest signal, which is obtained by placing the transducer over the location of the fetal heart
8. Adjust the audio-volume control while moving the transducer over the abdomen	8. To obtain the strongest fetal signal
9. Secure the ultrasound transducer with the abdominal belt or other fixation device	9. To prevent displacement of transducer

Procedure	Rationale
10. Observe the indicator signal, which will flash simultaneously with each fetal heartbeat	10. To verify clarity of input and ensure correct placement of the transducer
11. Set the recorder at 3 cm/min* paper speed and observe the FHR on the strip chart; obtain the baseline FHR *between* contractions or periodic changes	11. To ensure that paper feeds correctly and that recording is clear
12. Check the time printed on the monitor strip (reset monitor clock as necessary)	12. To ensure that the monitor prints out the accurate time
13. Periodically clean the transducer and maternal abdomen with a damp cloth to remove dried gel; reapply ultrasonic coupling gel and use talcum powder to dust under the abdominal belt if this is the fixation device	13. To keep the skin dry and promote the patient's comfort
14. Reposition the transducer whenever the fetal signal becomes unclear, such as when the mother moves or when the fetus descends in the pelvis	14. To ensure a clear, interpretable tracing during fetal monitoring

Advantages of the ultrasound transducer

- Noninvasive
- Easy to apply
- May be used during the antepartum period
- Does not require ruptured membranes or cervical dilatation
- No known hazards to mother or fetus
- Provides continuous recording of FHR
- Provides permanent record of FHR

*1 to 2 cm/min is used in some countries.

- Can differentiate FHR from maternal heart rate (eliminating errors caused by displacement)

Limitations

- Limits maternal movement
- Requires repositioning with fetal or maternal position change that results in loss of signal
- Can assess only relative short-term variability
- May double-count a slow FHR of less than 60 bpm (because of the inability to distinguish the first from the second heart sound so that they are both counted as equals)*
- May half-count a tachyarrhythmia of more than 180 bpm (because of the inability to reset, which can result in the skipping or elimination of every other heartbeat)*
- Maternal heart rate may be counted if the ultrasound transducer is placed over the maternal arterial vessels, such as the aorta
- Obese patients may be difficult to monitor because of the distance between the transducer and the fetal heart

Abdominal ECG transducer

The abdominal ECG transducer is capable of obtaining the FHR through the maternal abdominal wall. However, it is rarely used because of the time required to obtain an interpretable tracing as a result of fastidious skin preparation and electrode placement. The advantages of the ultrasound transducer far outweigh the utility of the abdominal ECG. The use of this technique has virtually disappeared.

Tocotransducer (tocodynamometer)
Description

The tocotransducer monitors uterine activity transabdominally by means of a pressure-sensing button that is depressed by uterine contractions or fetal movement. The uterine activity panel of the chart paper displays relative frequency and duration of contractions. Intensity and resting tone can be assessed only with the intrauterine catheter. The tocotransducer can be used to monitor uterine activity during both the antepartum and intrapartum periods.

---

*Auscultation can verify monitor double/half count.

General Guidelines for Care and Storage of External Transducers

- Exercise caution when handling the ultrasound and tocotransducers so that they are not dropped or allowed to swing against any equipment, to protect from damage.
- Clean transducers according to the manufacturer's operating manual, usually with a soft cloth using mild soap and water. Avoid submerging transducers or placing them underneath running water. Do not use alcohol or other cleaning solutions that will damage the equipment.
- Gently and loosely coil cables and secure with a rubber band for storage. Avoid tight coiling and sharp bending of the cables, which will result in damage to the wires or casing.
- Cables between monitor models and manufacturers are usually not interchangeable. Forced insertion into an inappropriate monitor will likely result in damage and render the equipment inoperable.
- Dispose of disposable abdominal belts. Wash reusable belts according to the facility's or manufacturer's suggested procedure before the next patient's use.

The procedure and rationale for the application of the tocotransducer is provided in a sequential format below.

Procedure	Rationale
1. Explain the procedure to the patient and her family	1. To allay anxiety
2. Gather the necessary equipment: fetal monitor, tocotransducer (tocodynamometer), and the equipment desired to monitor the FHR	2. To ensure that all equipment is readily accessible

Procedure	Rationale
3. Position the abdominal belt around the patient's upper abdomen, over the upper uterine segment, and place her in a semilateral position of comfort	3. To avoid supine hypotension syndrome
4. Perform Leopold's maneuvers (see Appendix B)	4. To determine fetal position
5. Align and insert the toco-transducer plug into the appropriate monitor port labeled "UA" (for uterine activity) or "Toco"	5. To provide connection without damaging connector pins, which could result in a faulty signal
6. Place the transducer on the maternal abdomen over the upper uterine segment where there is the least amount of maternal tissue between the pressure-sensing button and the uterus (where uterine contractions are best palpated)	6. To ensure that the upper uterine segment is as close as possible to the pressure-sensing button
7. Secure the tocotransducer with the abdominal belt and ensure that there is no gel under the tocotransducer	7. To prevent displacement of the transducer and to ensure that there is no damage to the tocotransducer from accumulation of gels
8. Set the recorder at 3 cm/min* paper speed, check the printed time/date for accuracy, and observe the strip chart	8. To ensure that the paper feeds correctly and that recording is clear

*1 to 2 cm/min is used in some countries.

Procedure	Rationale
9. Press the UA or Toco test button and adjust the sensitivity calibration device between contractions to print at the 20 mm Hg line on the chart paper	9. To prevent missing the very beginning or ending of the uterine contraction, which is necessary for FHR pattern interpretation
10. Monitor the frequency and duration of the contractions and document them in the patient's flow chart according to facility policy	10. The tocotransducer *cannot* measure intensity of contractions or resting tone between contractions because the depression of the pressure-sensing button varies with the amount of maternal adipose tissue; therefore the information should not be relied on to assess need for analgesia in relation to strength (painfulness) of contractions as registered by the monitor
11. When monitoring is in progress, readjust the abdominal strap periodically, and massage any reddened skin areas; a small amount of powder can be applied under the belt	11. To promote comfort and maintain the proper position of the transducer
12. Palpate the fundus every 30 to 60 minutes; *do not* rely on "peak pressure" of contraction to determine need for analgesia or titration of oxytocin	12. To assess relative pressure of contraction, because tocotransducer can relate only frequency and duration of contractions; it cannot assess intensity or resting tone
13. Reposition the transducer periodically and secure the abdominal belt snugly	13. To promote and ensure a good recording

Advantages of the tocotransducer

- Noninvasive
- Does not require ruptured membranes or cervical dilatation
- Is easily applied
- May be used with telemetry
- Provides continuous recording of contraction frequency and duration

Limitations

- Information is limited to frequency and duration
- Cannot assess strength or intensity of contractions
- Periodic repositioning of transducer may be necessary
- Limits patient's mobility
- May not get an interpretative tracing from an obese patient

Internal Mode of Monitoring
Spiral electrode
Description

The spiral electrode monitors the fetal ECG from the presenting part. It can be applied only after the membranes are ruptured, when the cervix is 2 to 3 cm or more dilated, and when the presenting part is accessible and identifiable (Figure 3-6). Therefore the spiral electrode can be used only during the intrapartum period. Use of

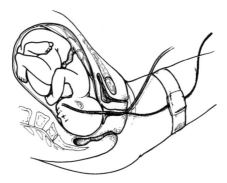

Figure 3-6
Diagrammatic representation of internal mode of monitoring with intrauterine catheter and spiral electrode in place.

the spiral electrode is contraindicated in patients suspected of having active herpes, HIV, or when there is vaginal bleeding and placenta previa has not been ruled out.

A sequential format for use of the spiral electrode is provided below.

Procedure	Rationale
1. Explain the procedure to the patient and her family	1. To allay anxiety
2. Gather necessary equipment: disposable spiral electrode, leg plate with cable, leg plate strap, and electrode paste	2. To ensure that all equipment is readily accessible
3. Position the leg plate strap around the woman's thigh, securing the leg plate to the thigh	3. To ensure transmission of electrical signal
4. Turn the power on and insert the cable into the appropriate monitor port labeled "ECG" or "Cardio"	4. To connect cable plug to appropriate outlet

5. Assist the physician, nurse midwife, or nurse in performing a sterile vaginal examination in order to apply the spiral electrode*
  a. Insert the entire apparatus through the vagina and cervix against the fetal presenting part
  b. Rotate the inner tube clockwise one full turn until gentle resistance is encountered
  c. Remove and discard the outer drive tube
	5. The electrode must be securely attached to ensure a good signal; the fetal face, fontanels, and genitals are avoided, and the electrode penetrates the skin of the presenting part 1.5 mm

*Registered nurses may insert the spiral electrode if this is allowed by licensing board regulations and if the nurse is credentialled and approved by the institutions policies.

Procedure	Rationale
6. Connect to the disposable leg plate pad or attach the color-coded wires to the appropriate posts on the reusable leg plate	6. To provide proper polarity for ECG tracing
7. Observe the indicator light, which will flash simultaneously with each fetal heartbeat	7. To verify clear signal from electrode
8. Set the recorder at 3 cm/min* paper speed, and observe the FHR on the strip chart	8. To ensure that the paper feeds correctly and that the recording is clear
9. Depress the test button for 10 seconds and make a notation of this on the strip chart; ensure that the monitor clock reflects the accurate time	9. To ensure that the monitor prints out a predetermined number (usually 120 or 150 bpm) on the corresponding line of the chart paper according to the manufacturer's guidelines in the operating manual
10. During monitoring check the leg plate periodically, and reposition for comfort as needed NOTE: The spiral electrode must be moist in vaginal secretions or signal transmission may be impaired	10. To ensure transmission of the signal
11. When removing the spiral electrode, turn 1½ turns counterclockwise or until it is free from the fetal presenting part; do not pull the electrode from the fetal skin; disconnect the elec-	11. To ensure that the electrode is removed in the same manner that it is applied; pulling the electrode straight out results in unnecessary trauma to the fetal skin, produces an observable

*1 to 2 cm/min paper speed is used in some countries.

Procedure	Rationale
trode from the leg plate and dispose of electrode appropriately NOTE: The electrode should be removed just before cesarean delivery and should not be left attached and brought up through the uterine incision. If unable to detach, cut wire at perineum and notify physician	wound, and predisposes the site to infection
12. Remove the leg strap and dispose of it, if it is disposable, or wash if it is reusable	12. To ensure that the disposable belt is not reused and that the reusable belt is cleaned and ready for future use
13. Clean the reusable leg plate according to the facility's procedure, or follow the manufacturer's directions in the operating manual	13. To prevent infection
14. Loosely coil the cable and secure with a rubber band, or place loosely coiled in a secure area	14. To prevent damage to the wires, which can occur with tight coiling, resulting in loss of or an inadequate fetal signal
15. Clean the fetal insertion site with a povidone-iodine swab unless otherwise directed by hospital policy or procedure	15. To prevent infection

Advantages of the spiral electrode

- Can assess both long- and short-term variability
- Positional changes do not affect quality of tracing
- Can accurately display fetal cardiac arrhythmias
- Accurately displays FHR between 30 and 240 bpm
- Is more comfortable than external transducer belt

Limitations

- Membranes must be ruptured
- Cervix must be dilated at least 2 cm
- Presenting part must be accessible and identifiable
- Need moist environment for FHR detection (difficult to monitor when fetal head is crowning)
- May record maternal heart rate (with fetal demise)
- May miss fetal arrhythmias if logic or ECG activation switch is engaged

Intrauterine (transcervical) pressure catheter
Description

The intrauterine pressure catheter* monitors contraction frequency, duration, intensity, and resting tone (Figure 3-7). A small catheter is introduced vaginally (transcervically) into the uterus after the cervix is dilated 2 to 3 cm or sufficiently to identify the presenting part and the fetal membranes have been ruptured. The catheter is compressed during uterine contractions, placing pressure on a strain gauge, or pressure transducer. The pressure is then reflected on the tracing or strip chart in the form of mm Hg pressure.

Some internal pressure catheters have the pressure-sensing device within the catheter tip or cable. These do not require the instillation of sterile water for use. These catheters are provided with an amnioport (Intran Plus IUP-400, Koala) to allow simultaneous amniofusion and uterine activity monitoring.

Procedure	Rationale
1. Explain the procedure to the patient and her family	1. To allay anxiety
2. Gather necessary equipment: disposable intrauterine kit, sterile gloves, and other equipment to perform a sterile vaginal examination	2. To ensure that all equipment is readily accessible
3. Turn the power on and insert the reusable cable into	3. To activate the pressure transducer

*The intrauterine catheter is referred to as an *intrauterine pressure transducer (IUPT)* in some countries.

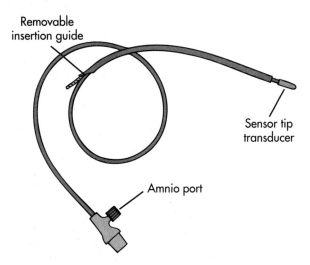

Figure 3-7
Intrauterine catheter with the sensor transducer located in the tip of the catheter provides uninterrupted uterine activity monitoring. Saline-filled catheters are another type of catheter in use. Note that this catheter has an amnioport that may be used for an amnioinfusion.

Procedure	Rationale
the appropriate monitor connector labeled "UA," "Toco," or "Utero"	
4. Before inserting a "fluid-filled catheter," fill the catheter with 5 ml sterile water, leaving the syringe attached to the catheter; maintain sterility of the maternal end of the catheter	4. To ensure that the catheter is patent and fluid-filled before insertion; to maintain aseptic technique
5. Prepare the patient/assist with a sterile vaginal examination; identify the fetal presenting part	5. To maintain aseptic technique and to identify the optimal location for catheter insertion

Procedure	Rationale
6. Insert the sterile catheter and introducer guide inside the cervix between the examining fingers; do not extend introducer guide beyond fingertips	6. The guide is made of a very hard plastic that can cause trauma if inserted farther than necessary
7. Advance only the catheter according to the insertion depth indicator or until the blue/black or stop mark on it reaches the vaginal introitus*	7. To ensure that enough of the catheter is inside the uterus; approximately 30 to 45 cm
8. Separate and remove or slide the catheter introducer guide away from the introitus and remove; dispose of guide appropriately	8. To prevent the guide from sliding toward the introitus
9. Secure the catheter to the patient's leg (for fluid-filled catheters, see p. 44)	9. To ensure patient mobility without fear of dislodging the catheter
10. Zero the monitor before connecting the catheter to the cable according to monitor manufacturer's instructions	10. To establish a zero baseline for the catheter system
11. Encourage patient to cough	11. To confirm a sharp spike on uterine activity tracing
12. Rezero monitor if indicated during labor	12. To ensure that uterine activity information is correct
13. Gently remove catheter after use and discard; store reusable cable for future use	13. To ensure that disposable catheter is not reused

*Remove catheter immediately in the event of *extraovular* placement outside of the amniotic fluid space (between the chorionic membrane and endometrial lining), as evidenced by blood in the catheter.

Perform the following procedures *only* for fluid-filled catheters:

Procedure	Rationale
a. Test or calibrate the strain gauge according to the manufacturer's instructions	a. To validate that uterine activity information is correct
b. Keeping the stopcock "Off" position pointed to the strain gauge, flush the catheter with 5 ml sterile water	b. To ensure that the catheter is patent and completely filled with fluid
c. Rotate the stopcock lever so that the "Off" position points to the catheter	c. To exclude pressure to the strain gauge
d. Release the pressure valve on the strain gauge and inject water from the syringe through the stopcock and gauge until all air bubbles are removed	d. To ensure that the strain gauge is completely filled with fluid
e. Release the pressure relief valve and then remove the syringe from the stopcock, maintaining its sterility	e. To open the system to atmospheric pressure
f. Press the record button; observe the tracing, which should print on the zero line of the uterine activity section of the chart paper; Adjust, or "zero," the pressure to ensure that the pen reads at the zero line of the monitor tracing	f. To verify that the tracing prints out on the zero line in the absence of pressure
g. Reattach the syringe to the stopcock; rotate the stopcock lever so that the "Off" position is pointing to the syringe; the uterine pressure system is now ready for monitoring	g. The solid column of water places pressure on the diaphragm of the strain gauge when it is compressed by uterine contractions; this results in an inflection on the uterine activity section of the strip chart in mm Hg

Procedure	Rationale
h. When monitoring is in progress:	
(1) Flush the intrauterine catheter with sterile water every 2 hours or as necessary (the use of solutions other than sterile water can occlude and corrode the system)	(1) To remove any vernix caseosa or air bubbles that may have entered the catheter and can invalidate the pressure reading
(2) Check the proper functioning of the catheter when necessary by tapping the catheter, asking the patient to cough, or applying fundal pressure while observing the chart	(2) To ensure inflection on the chart paper
i. Zero the catheter and test according to the manufacturer's directions	i. To ensure that the monitor traces on the appropriate line; this validates the accuracy of subsequent internal pressure monitoring
j. Apply gentle traction to remove catheter and dispose of catheter appropriately	j. To ensure that disposable equipment is not reused

Advantages of the intrauterine catheter

- Less confining and more comfortable than external mode of uterine activity monitoring
- Only accurate measure of uterine activity (e.g., frequency, duration, intensity, and resting tone)
- May be used with telemetry
- Records accurately regardless of maternal position
- Allows for an amnioinfusion to dilute meconium or treat variable decelerations that are uncorrected with traditional interventions

Limitations

- Membranes must be ruptured and cervix sufficiently dilated (e.g., 2 to 3 cm)

- Improper insertion can cause maternal or placental trauma
- Increased risk of infection

Troubleshooting the Monitor

The electronic fetal monitor is a useful tool to assess fetal well-being. As with any electronic device, problems may occur that can often be overcome. The following section suggests actions for identified problems.

Problem	Action
Power	■ Check power cord at wall and back of monitor
	■ Push in both ends of cord to ensure a tight fit (it may appear intact, although it is not)
Sixty-cycle interference	■ Check FHR by auscultation
	■ If there is improper grounding at the outlet or plug or in the machine, change to another electrical outlet, switch cords, or change electrode wires (on ground cable)
	■ Change electrode or monitor
Ultrasound Half or double rate	■ Assess FHR with fetoscope, stethoscope, or Doppler
	■ Check maternal pulse to rule out maternal signal and document maternal pulse
	■ Consider applying spiral electrode, or call physician to apply electrode if membranes are intact and bradycardia is present
	■ Reapply coupling gel and recheck
	■ Move transducer to search for a better signal
Intermittent ultrasound signal	■ Check ultrasound transducer: hold transducer by cord, allow transducer to hang, turn up volume, swing ultrasound transducer in the air; if static is heard, replace transducer; apply label to

Problem	Action
	broken transducer for repair or replacement
	■ Tighten belt if loose
	■ Check cable insertion site for a tight fit
Intermittent or no signal	■ Check gel on transducer; it may be dry (when gel is dry, sound waves do not penetrate the skin); reapply gel; move transducer if fetus is out of range
Direct FHR monitoring with spiral electrode	
Intermittent signal (individual dots on monitor strip or no signal)	■ Perform vaginal examination; check electrode placement; if loose, replace electrode
	■ Check that reference electrode is in vaginal secretions (instill fluid if necessary)
	■ Check ground cable on leg for adherence to skin
	■ Ensure that connection of electrode is secure on disposable leg plate pad or that color-coded wires are securely attached to the appropriate posts on the reusable leg plate
Signal and recording with stillborn (maternal signal is conducted through the stillborn infant)	■ Check and document maternal pulse (radial)
	■ Check with Doppler ultrasound device and suggest (or perform if qualified) ultrasound imaging to check for heart motion
Tocodynamometer (toco)	
No recording	■ Readjust toco on patient
Numbers in high range	■ Turn down the setting to a lower number on toco channel (if numbers cannot be turned down, toco needs repair); replace with another toco

Problem	Action
Toco not picking up contractions	■ Palpate abdomen for best quality of contractions and reapply toco
	■ Tighten belt, or use another device to hold toco firmly against abdomen
	■ Consider using intrauterine pressure catheter (IUPC) if patient is significantly obese
Intrauterine pressure catheter (IUPC)	
Not recording	■ Recheck cable insertion
Resting tone (≥ 20 mm Hg)	■ Adjust level of strain gauge for fluid-filled catheters
	■ Flush fluid-filled catheter
	■ Zero recalibrate non–fluid-filled catheter
Not recording contractions	■ Check catheter markings at patient's introitus (catheter may have slipped out)
	■ Replace catheter if necessary
High resting tone	■ Higher resting tone may be noted for: Oxytocin (20 mm Hg) Twins (30 mm Hg) Amnionitis (30 to 40 mm Hg)
	■ Decrease/discontinue oxytocin in presence of uterine hyperstimulation
Other problems	
Arrhythmia (occurs in 5% of pregnancies)	■ Turn up volume (can arrhythmia be heard?)
	■ Consult with other health professionals
	■ Check for variability, tachycardia, and bradycardia
	■ Auscultate FHR with fetoscope or stethoscope
	■ Perform fetal ECG
Errors caused by incorrect paper speed or monitor paper with different scale	■ Check annotation with paper speed; it should be 3 cm/min in North America
	■ Check scale; it should be 30 to 240 bpm for FHR if paper speed is 3 cm/min

Display of Fetal Heart Rate, Uterine Activity, and Other Information

The display on the front of the monitor includes FHR, with dual heart rates for twin gestations on some monitors, uterine pressure, and identification of the signal source for each. In addition there are various options available on monitors that can include maternal noninvasive blood pressure (NBP), maternal heart rate, maternal pulse oximetry ($MSpO_2$), maternal pulse rate obtained either by $MSpO_2$ or NPB, maternal ECG in real time, gross fetal body movements, and fetal oxygen saturation ($FSpO_2$). These parameters are also displayed on the front or face of the monitor.

The FHR and uterine activity (UA) are printed on scaled paper. The FHR is printed on the upper section and the uterine activity on the lower section (Figure 3-8). The following contrasts the FHR and uterine activity scaling systems used both domestically in the United States and internationally in the European community, Pacific Rim, and other areas.

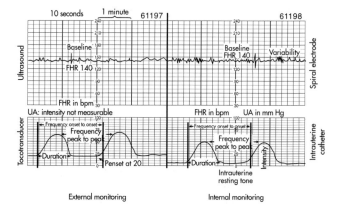

Figure 3-8

Display of FHR and uterine activity on monitor strip.
A, External mode of monitoring with ultrasound and tocotransducer. **B,** Internal mode of monitoring with spiral electrode and intrauterine catheter. Other significant information is supplied.

Fetal Monitor Paper Scale (Figure 3-9)

Axis	North America	Other Countries
Vertical Axis		
Heart Rate		
■ Range	30 to 240 bpm	50 to 210 bpm
■ Scale	30 bpm/cm increment	20 bpm/cm increment
Uterine Activity		
■ Range	0 to 100 mm Hg pressure	0-100 mm Hg pressure or 0 to 13.3 kilopascal units (1 kPa = 7.5 mm Hg)
■ Scale	5 or 10 mm Hg increments	10 mm Hg increments
Horizontal Axis		
■ Paper/recorder speed	3 cm/min = six 10-second subsections within 1 minute	1 cm/min = 2 subsection or 2 cm/min = 4 sub-sections

Monitors are preset by the manufacturers for the countries in which they are used; however, they can be changed if necessary. It is imperative to use the correctly scaled paper to match the domestic (3 cm/min) versus international (1 cm/min) monitor settings. For example, if domestic scaled paper is used and the monitor is set for international use, the FHR baseline rate will visually widen and the height and depth of periodic changes will increase.

Other parameters may be printed in addition to printing the FHR and UA on the tracing or strip chart. The time of day, date, and paper speed are usually printed every 10 minutes. The monitoring mode is usually printed every 3 to 4 pages of the tracing and with each change of parameter and mode of monitoring. Based on the monitor's options, other maternal and fetal data may be printed on the tracing. The maternal heart rate and maternal ECG can be trended on the upper heart rate section of the paper. The fetal oxygen saturation can be trended on the lower or uterine activity section of the paper. Some monitors have the capability of trending maternal oxygen saturation ($MSpO_2$) on the lower section of the tracing or printing it as whole numbers after each measurement. Noninvasive maternal blood pressure (NBP) can also be printed as whole numbers.

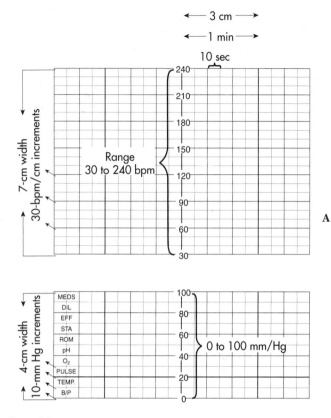

Figure 3-9

A, Fetal monitor paper scale: 3 cm/min speed used in North America with scaling information.   *Continued*

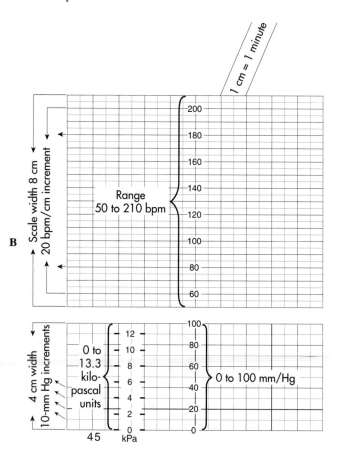

Figure 3-9, cont'd
B, Fetal monitor paper scale: 1 cm/min speed used in other countries with scaling information.

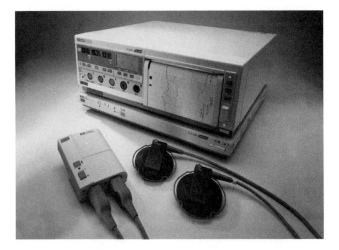

Figure 3-10
Telemetry unit underneath Viridia 50XM fetal monitor.
(Courtesy Agilent Technologies, Böblingen, Germany.)

The current time and signal source are also automatically printed on the trace or strip chart by some monitors. The manufacturer's operating manual should be available and referred to for more information, especially when assessing high-risk patients who may have concurrent monitoring of multiple parameters.

Telemetry

Remote internal or external FHR monitoring via radio wave telemetry (Figure 3-10) helps patients to remain ambulatory without the loss of continuous monitoring data. The patient may feel less confined, more relaxed, and more content if she can walk around. The transducer is worn by the patient by means of a shoulder strap or other device (Figure 3-11). Heart rate and uterine activity signals are continuously transmitted to a receiver that is connected to the fetal monitor. The monitor then processes the data, displays, and prints the heart rate and uterine activity on the strip chart. The telemetry unit should be connected to a fetal monitor that is hardwired to the central display in order to ensure surveillance by clinicians.

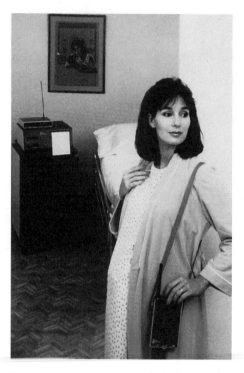

Figure 3-11
Ambulatory patient being monitored with telemetry unit.
(Courtesy GE Marquette Medical Systems, Milwaukee, Wis.)

In addition to the use of standard ultrasound and tocotransducers, watertight transducers are available. These can be used to continue fetal surveillance underwater. For example, the watertight transducers can be used with a wireless telemetry device when the patient is in a shower, spa, or bathtub.

In addition to the benefits of freedom of movement during labor and continuous monitoring within the labor suite or to the delivery room, telemetry has been applied in the outpatient setting for patients instructed to remain at rest in their own homes. Data from the transmitter can be sent via modem to the receiver unit, which is connected to a printer, producing a hard copy of the FHR strip chart. This transmission of information from the patient to the re-

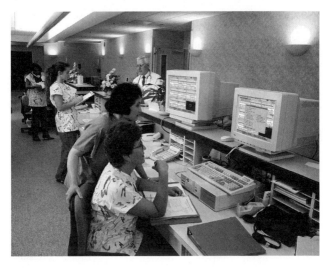

Figure 3-12
Patient care staff at a central station monitoring multiple patients.
(Courtesy GE Marquette Medical Systems, Milwaukee, Wis. Photograph by Jim Fiora.)

ceiver unit allows the clinician to determine the patient's status. Based on the data received, the patient's tocolytic needs may be adjusted, and consultation can be made with a referral center by the clinician to receive an expert's interpretation of the data.

Central Display

A central monitor display at the nurses' station provides an opportunity to view tracings from several patients at the same time (Figure 3-12). In addition, single-screen display of several patients can be accessed from remote locations, including the patient's bedside, staff locker room or lounge areas, a physician's office, or home. This can provide the staff with instant access to the patient's monitor pattern from any location and is especially important when the nurse cannot be in constant attendance. Some systems include the capability of data entry in the form of detailed notes about results of examinations, cervical dilatation, fetal station, administration of drugs, patient's position, and vital signs, all related to time. Reports may be generated with the integration of an optional printer linked to the display, which can contain complete patient information, history, and a graphic printout of the labor curve progression, providing a single and comprehensive document.

Some central display systems (Figure 3-13) can provide additional information, including the following:

1. A system status screen provides an instant overview of several beds on the system and indicates any alerts by room number. In addition, it can identify the signal source of any of the patients on the system.
2. A trend screen, which can provide the most recent past few minutes of heart rate and uterine activity data on any one patient, with immediate warning of critical conditions relating to any patient in the system.

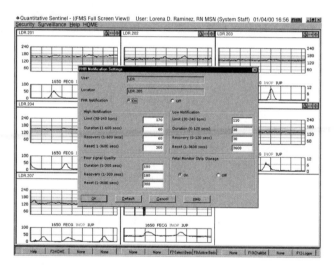

Figure 3-13
The QS-Surveillance allows the user to set the high/low ranges that will initiate an audible or visual notification for fetal bradycardia and tachycardia. If the heart rate violates the set limits and duration, the notification will continue until it has been acknowledged, even if the heart rate returns to an acceptable level. High/low ranges may be set at different levels for each patient.
(Courtesy GE Marquette Medical Systems, Milwaukee, Wis.)

3. An alert screen, which provides an immediate summary of the trend analysis on any patient. The data can be made available to the staff before, during, and after an alert.

Information Systems

Information systems combine fetal surveillance and alerting with patient documentation and data storage in one system that can cover the entire continuum of obstetrical care across several pregnancies. The *surveillance* component of the system can be set to alert for fetal tachycardia or bradycardia, signal loss, coincidental fetal and maternal heart rates, and all maternal and other parameters. Ranges for the duration and recovery from fetal bradycardia or tachycardia can be set at different levels for each patient.

In addition to improving the quality of care through surveillance and alert capabilities, another benefit to having a system that is accessible across the health care continuum, especially when integrated with other hospital or outpatient information systems, is to provide a database for statistical reporting for administration, research, and quality purposes. These systems can provide multiple data entry points across the continuum of care and among multiple campuses of a hospital network (Kelly, 1999). These points include the physician's office (Figure 3-14), ambulatory care clinic, antepartum testing center, inpatient department, labor and delivery suite or birthing center, and home health or continuing care department. For example, if a patient presents to the birthing center in the middle of the night, the staff can readily access the entire antenatal record, home uterine monitoring documents and the ultrasound, Non-Stress Test, or biophysical profile that was just completed the previous afternoon, even if it was at a different campus within the system.

Documentation on forms and flow sheets together with annotated tracings can provide complete electronic patient records and provide fast and easily retrievable information. The *archival* and *retrieval* of the original fetal monitoring tracing or strip has proved to be a problem for most medical record departments because the process is labor intensive and the paper space consuming. Microfiche records are less bulky to store but still take time to log, sort, and file in the medical record, although many facilities continue to do this. A welcome alternative has been computer-based storage systems on the hard drive and optical laser disks. These systems

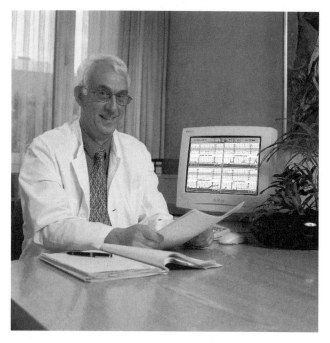

Figure 3-14
Physician can access FHR tracing in medical office.
(Courtesy Agilent Technologies, Böblingen, Germany.)

are best installed with a security system that prevents alteration or removal of the documents and a backup system in the event that there is damage or loss of the optical disk cartridge.

The ability to have multiple points of data entry, information retrieval, and reproduction of the patient's record and fetal monitor tracing is a significant advancement. This coupled with an interface to the hospital admission, discharge, and transfer (ADT) information system and other hospital-based information systems should contribute to the trend toward comprehensive, paperless, and fully electronic information systems.

Data Input Devices

Data input devices are an option with electronic fetal monitors and monitoring systems. Some of the options include use of a bar-code

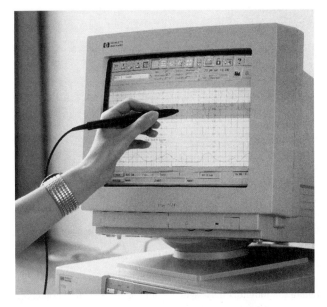

Figure 3-15
With color icons one can enter and access information
quickly and easily with a light pen, mouse, or keyboard.
(Courtesy Agilent Technologies, Böblingen, Germany.)

reader, key pads for data entry, light pens (Figure 3-15), touch
screens, remote event markers, and standard keyboards. The input
is subsequently printed on the tracing (Figure 3-16). The use of
these options can promote accurate documentation and help eliminate the need for handwritten annotations, which are sometimes il-
legible. In addition, information may be entered on the strip chart
automatically, including time (every 10 minutes), date, paper
speed, and monitoring mode.

Artifact Detection

Fetal monitors have built-in artifact rejection systems, which are always in operation when using the external mode of FHR monitoring. Logic circuitry rejects data when there is a greater variation
than is expected between successive fetal heartbeats. If there are repetitive variations by more than the accepted amount, the older-

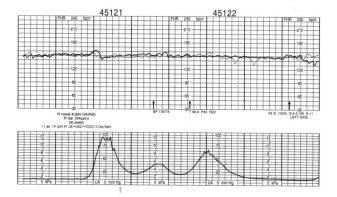

Figure 3-16
Tracing demonstrates pertinent data that has been entered
via a data input device.
(Courtesy GE Marquette Medical Systems, Milwaukee, Wis.)

generation monitors may switch from a hold mode to a nonrecord
mode (exhibited by penlift or no heat to the stylus). The recorder
resumes recording when the variation between successive beats
falls within the predetermined parameters. The newer monitors continue to print regardless of the extent of the excursion of the FHR.

During internal monitoring, artifact is rare, and the logic system
will miss only those changes that exceed the predetermined limits
of the system. If there is an accessible switch to select a logic or
no-logic mode, it is preferable to have the monitor in the no-logic
mode when using the internal mode (spiral electrode) in order to
detect fetal arrhythmias. When recording internally, the logic-on
should be used only when there is true artifact, such as with poor
signal-to-noise ratio (caused by extraneous electrical noise), or
when there is a large maternal R wave that is counted on an intermittent basis. This can usually be determined by printing out the
fetal ECG.

Considerations Before Monitor Purchase

Various monitors are available, and generally they have the same
capabilities. In considering a monitor for purchase, however, it is
prudent to use the desired model on a trial basis and to consult with
people who have used the type of equipment being considered

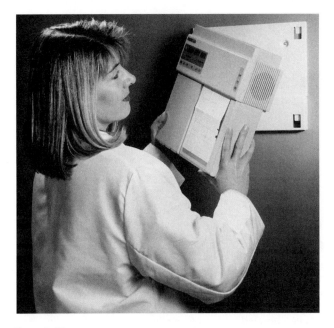

Figure 3-17
Space-saving designed HP Series 50 A and IP fetal monitors
are compact and lightweight and function equally well
mounted on a wall, table top, or mobile cart.
(Courtesy Agilent Technologies, Böblingen, Germany.)

(Figures 3-17 and 3-18). The following items should also be
considered:

1. Accuracy of data output
2. Ease of use
3. Reliability for continuous functioning with minimum down/
   repair time
4. Repair frequency and history from other facilities using the
   same monitor (turnaround time for service)
5. Cost of monitor and other expendable supplies (e.g., paper,
   abdominal belts)
6. Availability of expendable supplies from multiple sources for
   better cost advantage
7. Legible display and function labels

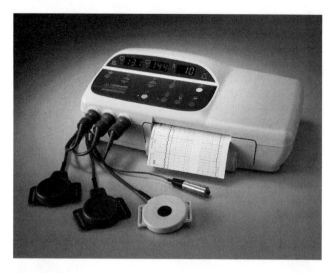

Figure 3-18
The Corometrics 170 Series noninvasive fetal monitor is a
compact, lightweight unit with single or dual ultrasounds
that can be used in the office, clinic, or hospital setting. This
monitor features a high/low heart rate alarm, telemetry
interface, fetal movement detection capability, and a FASt
(Fetal Acoustic Stimulator) interface.
(Courtesy GE Marquette Medical Systems. Photograph by Jim Fiora.)

8. Complexity of paper refill procedure
9. Training time needed for users or video training films included
   with purchase
10. Training services and support from the company at little or no
    cost
11. Fragility of ultrasound transducer, cable, and connectors
12. History and stability of company and frequency of changing
    models
13. Expected life of the equipment
14. Interchangeability of transducers from one model to the next
    within the same company (to avoid the possibility of built-in
    obsolescence)

Uterine Activity Monitoring

4

Methods: Palpation and Electronic Monitoring

Assessment of uterine activity (UA) includes the identification of contraction frequency, duration, and strength. Uterine activity can be assessed by manual palpation, or electronic monitoring with either external monitoring using a tocotransducer (tocodynamometer) or internal monitoring using an intrauterine pressure catheter (IUPC) (Figure 4-1).*

Palpation

Manual palpation has been the traditional method of monitoring contractions. This method can measure contraction frequency, duration, and relative strength. Palpation is a learned skill that is best performed with the fingertips to feel the uterus rise upward as the contraction develops. *Mild, moderate,* and *strong* are the terms used to describe what is felt by the examiner's hands during palpation and is based on the degree of indentation of the abdomen (AWHONN, 1997). For learning and comparison purposes the degree of indentation corresponds to the palpation sensation when feeling the parts of the adult face as described below.

Contraction Strength	Palpation Sensation
Mild	Tense fundus but easy to indent (feels like touching finger to tip of nose)
Moderate	Firm fundus, difficult to indent with fingertips (feels like touching finger to chin)

*The intrauterine pressure catheter is referred to as an *intrauterine pressure transducer (IUPT)* in some countries.

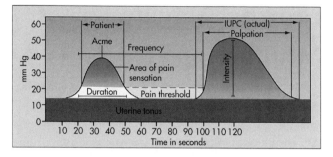

Figure 4-1
Comparison of relative sensitivity of assessing uterine
contractions by internal monitoring (IUPC), manual
palpation, and patient perception. External monitor is
variable.
(Modified from Dickason EJ, Silverman BL, Kaplan JA: *Maternal-infant nursing care,* ed 3, St Louis, 1998, Mosby.)

Contraction Strength	Palpation Sensation
Strong	Rigid, boardlike fundus, almost impossible to indent (feels like touching finger to forehead)

The majority of labors in the world are managed by palpation, which promotes maternal ambulation and freedom of movement. Palpation as the sole method of monitoring uterine activity is less frequent in hospitals in North America than in other countries. There are multiple factors that contribute to this practice.

Electronic Monitoring

Electronic monitoring provides continuous data and a permanent record of uterine activity. *External uterine activity monitoring* is achieved using a tocotransducer (tocodynamometer) to provide information on uterine contraction frequency and duration and a relative idea of strength. Because the contraction display depends on the depression of a pressure-sensing button placed on the maternal abdomen, there are variations in depression caused by placement location and the amount of maternal adipose tissue. For example, a thin patient may exhibit large inflections when having mild contractions, in contrast to an obese patient, who may exhibit minor inflections when having strong contractions. In addition, belt tightness, position of the tocotransducer, and maternal and fetal position can all greatly affect the recording of uterine activity. Therefore the strength of the uterine contraction must be assessed by manual palpation when uterine activity is externally monitored.

Internal uterine activity monitoring is achieved using an intrauterine pressure catheter that measures absolute intensity of the uterine contraction and resting tone in addition to contraction frequency and duration. The following list contrasts these two modes of monitoring.

	External Mode	Internal Mode
Signal source	Tocotransducer (tocodynamometer)	Intrauterine pressure catheter
Data	1. Frequency of contractions (measured from the onset of one contraction to the onset of the next contraction)	1. Frequency of contractions (measured from the onset of one contraction to the onset of the next contraction or from peak of one contraction to the peak of the next contraction if the contractions are bell shaped and not skewed)
	2. Duration of contractions (from beginning to end)	2. Duration of contractions (from beginning to end)
	3. Relative strength of contractions dependent on abdominal pressure against pressure-sensing device; the abdomen must be palpated to assess strength of contraction based on degree of indentation of the fundus	3. Intensity of contractions (mm Hg pressure at peak of contraction)

External Mode	Internal Mode
4. Resting tone (the abdomen must be palpated to assess resting tone based on the degree of indentation of the fundus)	4. Resting tone (mm Hg pressure between contractions)

Electronic display of uterine activity

Uterine activity is monitored and recorded on the lower section of the chart panel (Figure 4-2). The range of the scale is from 0 to 100 mm Hg pressure, with five major vertical sections of 20 mm Hg each, with each of the smaller lines in between representing 10 mm Hg. Some tracing paper used in North America has four major vertical sections of 25 mm Hg each, with the smaller lines representing 5 mm Hg pressure.

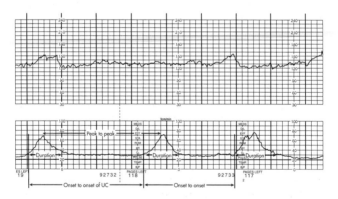

Figure 4-2
Frequency of uterine contractions can be measured from the onset of one UC to the onset of the next. Frequency can also be measured from the peak of one UC to the peak of the next *unless* the peak is skewed as it is on the third contraction.

Uterine Activity Progression and Quantitation

In a normal labor, uterine contractions occur about every 2 to 5 minutes, with a duration of 30 to 60 seconds and an increasing strength of uterine contractions from mild to moderate to strong over the course of the labor. When monitored internally, the intensity of the contractions can range from 30 to 80 mm Hg pressure, with a resting tone between 5 and 15 mm Hg. In addition to identifying this information, the chart panel also indicates fetal movement by "blips," spikes, or momentary increases in uterine pressure. Identification of fetal movement is important, because it forms the basis for antepartum nonstress testing by identifying fetal *reactivity,* or the presence of accelerations with fetal movement.

The use of a labor curve, also described as a *partogram* or *cervicograph,* may be used to graph the progress of labor and provides a visual means of recording cervical dilatation and station across the course of time (Figure 4-3). As the fetal presenting part descends and cervical dilatation increases, the lines cross each other in an X pattern. When the patient's progress is compared with a normal labor curve for the latent and active phases of labor, the identification of a normal, dysfunctional, or precipitous labor may become evident. Identification of dysfunctional labor is addressed in Appendix C, Protocols for the Initiation of Labor: Cervical Ripening, Amniotomy, and Oxytocin Augmentation/ Induction.

In addition to the use of a labor curve to monitor the progress of labor, Montevideo units (MVU) have been used as a quantitation measure of uterine activity. Calculation of MVU requires the use of an intrauterine pressure catheter. This method was described by Caldeyro-Barcia in 1957 as the product of the average contraction peak in mm Hg multiplied by the number of contractions in a 10-minute period (Caldeyro-Barcia, Poseiro, 1960). Another method of calculating MVU is to subtract the baseline intrauterine pressure (the resting tone) from the peak of the contraction pressure for each contraction in a 10-minute window. These numbers are then added together to determine the number of MVU (ACOG, 1995a). However, in clinical use the value is quickly and roughly obtained by adding the peak

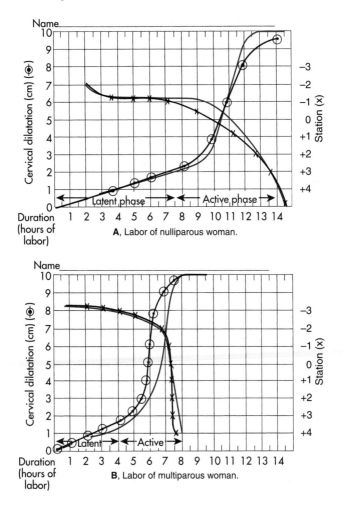

A, Labor of nulliparous woman.

B, Labor of multiparous woman.

Figure 4-3

Partogram for assessment of patterns of cervical dilatation and descent. Individual woman's labor patterns *(black)* superimposed on prepared labor graph for comparison. **A,** Labor of a nulliparous woman. **B,** Labor of a multiparous woman. The rate of cervical dilatation is plotted with the circled plot points. A line drawn through these symbols depicts the slope of the curve. Station is plotted with Xs. A line drawn through the Xs reveals the pattern of descent.

(Modified from Lowdermilk DL et al: *Maternity nursing,* ed 5, St Louis, 1999, Mosby.)

intensities of each contraction in a 10-minute period (Parer, 1997). Adequate uterine activity in labor is defined to be greater than 200 MVU. Although this quantitation measure has been used by investigators, it is limited by not including the duration of the contraction in the calculations.

Summary of Normal Uterine Activity Pattern

Frequency	More than 2 minutes between contractions
Duration	Contractions 30 to 60 seconds: less than 90 seconds
Intensity	Less than 80 mm Hg pressure
Resting tone	Thirty seconds or more between contractions; resting intrauterine pressure less than 20 mm Hg (can be determined only by intrauterine monitoring)

Increased Uterine Activity

During intrapartum monitoring of uterine activity, it is important to look for hyperstimulation of the uterus in addition to the frequency, duration, and intensity of contractions and intrauterine resting tone. Hyperstimulation, as evidenced by increased uterine activity on the chart panel, can result in a decrease in fetal oxygenation because of interference with the uteroplacental circulation. An outlined description of increased uterine activity follows.

Observations

1. Contractions lasting longer than 90 seconds
2. Relaxation between contractions less than 30 seconds
3. Inadequate intrauterine relaxation with resting tone above 20 mm Hg between contractions
4. Peak pressure of contractions above 80 mm Hg
5. Contractions more frequent than every 2 minutes

Causes

1. Hyperstimulation of the uterus with oxytocin
2. Abruptio placentae
3. Overdistension of the uterine wall as a result of multiple gestation, hydramnios, or a macrosomic fetus
4. Pregnancy-induced hypertension
5. Drugs
    a. Narcotics (e.g., meperidine hydrochloride [Demerol])
    b. Beta-blocking agents (e.g., propranolol [Inderal])
    c. Prostaglandins (e.g., prostaglandin E_2 alpha [$PGE_2\alpha$, Dinoprost])
    d. Pituitary hormones (e.g., vasopressin [Pitressin])
    e. Estrogen
    f. Ergonovine

Clinical Significance

Hyperstimulation of the uterus or hypertonus can result in stress to the fetus (as a result of the lack of placental perfusion) and potentially in uterine rupture. The most common cause of uterine hyperstimulation is the injudicious use of oxytocin. When an oxytocin infusion is discontinued, uterine relaxation usually occurs within 10 minutes, with return of normal baseline FHR and variability. When oxytocin is given by poorly controlled methods, such as the buccal or intramuscular route, there is an added risk because the rate of absorption and any adverse fetal effects are prolonged (Figure 4-4). A protocol for the administration of oxytocin for induction or augmentation of labor is in Appendix C.

Because uterine contractions are known to decrease the rate of blood flow through the intervillous space and most fetuses are well

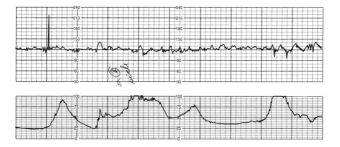

Figure 4-4
Uterine hyperstimulation from oxytocin.

able to tolerate this transient type of stress, it is important to atten-
tively monitor uterine activity in addition to FHR. In pregnancies
in which the margin of fetal reserve is low, this phenomenon can
cause commensurate decreases in FHR (described as *late decelerations*). The provider should be promptly notified when there is
evidence of uterine hyperstimulation with or without an associated
heart rate response.

Intervention

1. Discontinue oxytocin if infusing (exercise caution in flushing
   the oxytocin out of the line to ensure that a bolus is not delivered to the patient).
2. Increase rate of maintenance intravenous infusion.
3. Change maternal position (left lateral preferred).
4. Consider administration of oxygen, 8 to 10 L/min by face mask,
   depending on response in FHR.
5. Perform fetal scalp stimulation test to assess fetal well being
   (p. 137).
6. The provider may consider the use of tocolytics such as terbutaline or magnesium sulfate if there is an excessive increase
   in uterine activity, such as hypertonus, and a nonreassuring
   FHR pattern is evident.
   Fetal recovery from uterine hypertonus is preferred in utero because once the placental circulation is restored, carbon dioxide
from respiratory acidosis, as well as the acidic products of anaerobic metabolism, can be eliminated.

Inhibition of Uterine Activity
Tocolytics

It is important to decrease uterine activity when premature labor or nonreassuring FHR patterns occur. Drugs such as isoxsuprine, epinephrine, and isoproterenol have been used in the past to reduce uterine activity but not without drawbacks (i.e., their beta-stimulant effects cause vasodilation and secondary hypotension). Because of their extrauterine effects, beta-mimetic agents are now used. Terbutaline is now routinely used because it has maximal uterine relaxant effects. In addition, magnesium sulfate or nifedipine is frequently considered as the first choice in tocolytic therapy. Other drugs known to inhibit uterine activity include diazoxide, halothane, progesterone, and prostaglandin inhibitors (e.g., ibuprofen and indomethacin).

In the past, ethanol (alcohol) was widely used to successfully stop premature labor in some patients, but in others it had detrimental results. It is no longer used, however. Alcohol can depress maternal central respiratory and vasomotor centers, inducing secondary hypoxia.

See the box below for a list of drugs known to inhibit uterine activity. A protocol for the management of preterm labor can be found in Appendix D.

Drugs Inhibiting Uterine Activity

1. Beta-sympathomimetics (e.g., terbutaline and ritodrine)
2. Magnesium sulfate
3. Calcium-channel blockers (e.g., nifedipine)
4. Prostaglandin inhibitors (e.g., indomethacin)
5. Diazoxide
6. Ethanol
7. Halothane
8. Progesterone

Baseline Fetal Heart Rate

Since the advent and widespread use of electronic fetal monitoring, various descriptive terms have been used to describe fetal heart rate (FHR) patterns. The definitions of these terms have not always been globally consistent among practitioners and institutions, resulting in variation in interpretation of FHR tracings. In addition, this lack of standardization and consistency in definitions and nomenclature for FHR patterns has been an impediment to progress in the investigation and evaluation of FHR monitoring.

The National Institute of Child Health and Human Development (NICHD) brought together clinicians, experts in electronic fetal monitoring, from the United States, Canada, and the United Kingdom (NICHD, 1997). Their purpose was to standardize a clear set of definitions that could be quantitated, thus providing a foundation for electronic fetal monitoring terminology used in practice and research. Through the standardized definitions, the predictive value of monitoring can be assessed more meaningfully in appropriately designed observational studies and clinical trials. The hope is that the resulting research-based investigative interpretation will lead to a more evidence-based clinical management of FHR tracings.

The NICHD definitions were primarily developed for visual FHR interpretation but are intended to apply also to computerized interpretation. Definitions apply to FHR patterns produced from either a direct fetal electrode detecting the fetal electrocardiogram (FECG) or an external Doppler ultrasound device detecting the fetal heart events using the autocorrelation technique. Although the prime emphasis of the definitions is for intrapartum patterns, they are also applicable to antepartum observations. The NICHD definitions are used as a basis for the content in this book.

Baseline Fetal Heart Rate

Definition

Baseline FHR is the average (mean) FHR rounded to increments of 5 beats per minute (bpm) during a 10-minute segment of a tracing and excludes:

1. Periodic or episodic changes
2. Periods of marked FHR variability
3. Segments of the baseline which differ by >25 bpm

In any 10-minute segment, the minimum baseline duration must be at least 2 minutes, otherwise the baseline is considered to be indeterminate. In this case, the baseline FHR may then need to be determined from the previous 10-minute segment(s). The normal range of FHR at term is 110 to 160 bpm (NICHD, 1997).

Description

Baseline FHR is set by the atrial pacemaker and balanced by an interplay between the sympathetic (cardioaccelerator) and parasympathetic (decelerator) branches of the autonomic nervous system. As a result of immaturity of the central nervous system and the sympathetic dominance, the premature fetus at approximately 20 weeks' gestation may exhibit a baseline heart rate of 150 to 170 bpm. In the healthy full-term infant, the rate is usually between 110 and 160 bpm. This is the result of the balanced regulatory interaction between parasympathetic and sympathetic nervous systems. A fetus over the age of 40 weeks' gestation may have a rate between 110 and 120 bpm. This rate indicates a slightly greater influence of parasympathetic control.

Assessment of the baseline FHR can be facilitated during periods when there is no stress or stimuli to the fetus. The following guidelines may be used, especially when it is difficult to assess the baseline FHR (Figure 5-1):

1. When the patient is not in labor
2. When the fetus is not moving
3. Between uterine contractions
4. When there is no stimulation to the fetus as occurs with vaginal examinations and placement of an internal monitoring device
5. During the interval between periodic changes

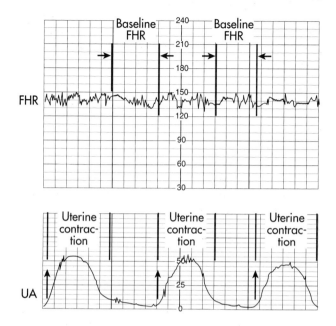

Figure 5-1
Baseline FHR is usually easier to assess between uterine contractions.

Variability
Definition

Baseline FHR variability is defined as fluctuations in the baseline FHR of 2 cycles per minute or greater. These fluctuations are irregular in amplitude and frequency and are visually quantitated as the amplitude of the peak-to-trough in beats per minute as follows (NICHD, 1997):

Descriptive Term (Figure 5-2)	Amplitude Range
Absent	1. Undetectable
Minimal	2. ≥ Undetected to ≤5 bpm
Moderate [average]	3. 6 to 25 bpm
Marked	4. >25 bpm

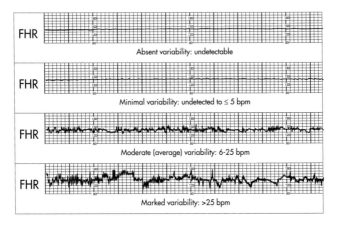

Figure 5-2
Classification of variability.

Description

Variability of the FHR can be described as the normal irregularity of cardiac rhythm, resulting from a continuous balancing interaction of the sympathetic (cardioacceleration) and parasympathetic (cardiodeceleration) branches of the autonomic nervous system. These two branches interact, modulating the FHR. Average variability of the FHR is demonstrated by fluctuations of the baseline, which reflect an intact neurological pathway, optimal fetal oxygenation, and the measure of fetal oxygen reserve in the tissue. In addition, intrapartum baseline variability indirectly indicates fetal tolerance of labor.

Variability is considered to be the most important FHR characteristic and reflects neurological modulation of the FHR. The fetus who exhibits moderate variability (reassuring) indicates a capability to centralize available oxygen and will remain physiologically compensated. If each interval between successive heartbeats were exactly the same, as in the regular rhythm of a ticking clock or metronome, the baseline would be flat, indicating central nervous system depression associated with hypoxia or a previous insult with some central nervous system impairment. Therefore absence of variability of the FHR is demonstrated by a smooth or flat baseline.

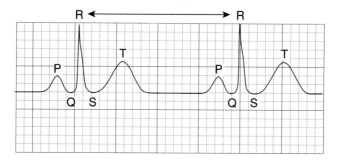

Figure 5-3
FHR tracings from a fetal spiral electrode are obtained by
fetal electrocardiogram (FECG) measuring the interval
between consecutive fetal R waves. A cardiotachometer
processes the interval between R waves to a rate in beats
per minute, which is printed on the monitor tracing. This
illustration demonstrates the time interval between R waves.
However, in the healthy fetus the intervals should vary,
showing *variability* in the FHR from one beat to the next.

In the NICHD definitions, no distinction is made between short-
term variability (STV) and long-term variability (LTV). In actual
practice, STV and LTV are viewed together and determined visually as a unit. In addition, the definition of variability excludes the
sinusoidal pattern discussed later in this chapter, because this pattern has a smooth sine wave of regular frequency and amplitude.

Although the definition for variability is objective and clear for
visual interpretation, the characteristics of STV and LTV can be
recognized. STV is the beat-to-beat change in FHR from one heartbeat to the next. STV is often described as present or absent. STV
reflects the internal difference between successive R peaks of the
FECG signal (Figure 5-3). It is a reflection of the normal irregularity in the interval between consecutive heartbeats (cardiac rhythm)
and is controlled by the parasympathetic nervous system. Direct
ECG (scalp electrode) is the only method that can accurately measure STV (ACOG, 1995d). STV is the sensitive indicator of fetal
oxygenation and oxygen reserve in the tissue. Presence of STV is
reassuring in that it indicates that the fetus appropriately responds
to nerve impulses and has an intact autonomic nervous system.

Table 5-1   Fetal heart rate variability

	Short Term	Long Term
Description	A change in FHR from one beat to the next "beat-to-beat"	Rhythmical and cyclical fluctuations in FHR of ≥ 2 cycles per minute
Appearance		
Signal source	Spiral electrode	Spiral electrode and ultrasound transducer

LTV is influenced by the sympathetic nervous system. LTV is the rhythmical fluctuations in FHR, excluding accelerations, decelerations, and any aberrant marks and artifacts (Table 5-1). Interpretation of LTV is made by visual examination of the rise and fall (amplitude) and frequency of changes in FHR within the baseline range. The frequency of amplitude can be identified by determining the number of instances (cycles) per minute or the number of times the FHR crosses over the imaginary line determined as the average (median) of the baseline range (AWHONN, 1997). The presence of LTV gives an indication of fetal oxygenation and the physiological ability to compensate for stress. The absence of LTV is a marker for fetal hypoxia and indicates the need for implementation of interventions that will attempt to improve fetal oxygenation.

Generally, STV and LTV tend to increase and decrease together. This is caused by the interplay between the parasympathetic and sympathetic nervous systems and their response to external and internal factors. There are also certain instances when STV and LTV exhibit changes independently from each other (Figure 5-4). For example, when a fetus is sleeping, STV may be present and LTV decreased. There are also fetal conditions that result in FHR patterns in which LTV is present but STV is absent, such as in the presence of fetal anemia. When evaluating STV and LTV, and determining whether variability is reassuring or nonreassuring, other factors should be considered, including gestational

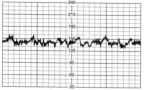

Both short- and
long-term variability

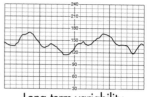

Long-term variability,
absence of short-term variability

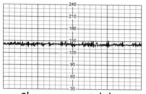

Short-term variability,
absence of long-term variability

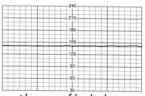

Absence of both short-
and long-term variability

Figure 5-4
Variations in short- and long-term variability.

age, drugs, stage of labor, anesthesia, obstetrical history, prenatal course, fetal condition, and the presence of fetal anomalies. These factors will help to determine the potential need for interventions.

The following section lists causes of increased and decreased variability with their clinical significance and potential interventions.

Cause of Variations in Variability	Clinical Significance/Intervention
Marked Variability	
1. Mild hypoxia An early compensatory mechanism produces an increase in short-term FHR variability	The significance of marked variability is not known. Marked or *saltatory* variability from a previous moderate (average) variability is thought to be a compensatory mechanism and an early sign of fetal hypoxia. Baseline variability should be evaluated before administration of medications. Unless deterior-
2. Fetal stimulation External uterine palpation, uterine contractions, fetal activity, application of spiral electrode, vaginal examination, acoustic	

Cause of Variations in Variability	Clinical Significance/Intervention
stimulation, and maternal activity stimulate the fetal autonomic nervous system, resulting in an increase in variability	ation of variability or a nonreassuring pattern develops, no intervention is required

3. Stimulant drugs
   Initial response is central nervous system excitability to cocaine, crack, and methamphetamines

4. Sympathomimetic drugs
   Terbutaline, ritodrine, and asthma medications; sympathetic response may cause maternal and fetal tachycardia in addition to increased variability

Decreased Variability

1. Hypoxia and acidosis Uteroplacental insufficiency as a result of several causes (uterine hyperstimulation, maternal supine hypotension, pregnancy-induced hypertension, amnionitis). (Other causes are listed under late decelerations.)	Decreasing variability is an indication of fetal stress. Absence of variability exhibited by a smooth or flat baseline is a significant sign of fetal distress. A flat or smooth baseline associated with late decelerations of *any* magnitude is a sign of advanced hypoxia and acidosis that is related to central nervous system depression. (Decreased variability related to drugs usually returns to previous baseline levels as the drug is excreted. If a central nervous system–depressant drug has been given near the time of delivery, Narcan may be administered to the neonate after delivery. Baseline variability should be evaluated before

Cause of Variations in Variability	Clinical Significance/Intervention
	administration of analgesics/narcotics and other drugs. Administration time and effect of drugs must be documented. Variability that is decreased as a result of fetal sleep patterns usually resumes in 20 to 30 minutes.) Efforts to improve and optimize fetal oxygenation and uteroplacental blood flow through maternal positioning, hydration, correction of maternal hypotension, maternal oxygenation, and elimination of uterine hyperstimulation are indicated. Application of a spiral electrode should be considered if the pattern is observed by external monitoring and the tracing is of poor quality
2. Drugs Narcotics, tranquilizers, barbiturates, and anesthetics depress central nervous system mechanisms responsible for cardiac control; anticholinergics such as atropine and scopolamine block the transmission of impulses to the sinoatrial node *Analgesics/narcotics* Meperidine hydrochloride (Demerol), morphine sulfate, heroin, methadone, nalbuphine hydrochloride (Nubain), butorphanol tartrate (Stadol), fentanyl, (Sublimaze)	Baseline variability should be evaluated before administration of analgesics/narcotics. Administration time and effect of medications given must be documented. Efforts to improve and optimize fetal oxygenation and uteroplacental blood flow through maternal positioning, hydration, correction of maternal hypotension, maternal oxygenation, and elimination of uterine hyperstimulation may be indicated. Application of a spiral electrode should be considered if the pattern is observed by external monitoring and the tracing is of poor quality

Cause of Variations in Variability	Clinical Significance/Intervention
Barbiturates Secobarbital sodium (Seconal), pentobarbital sodium (Nembutal), amobarbital (Amytal) *Anticonvulsant, uterine relaxant* Magnesium sulfate *Tranquilizers* Diazepam (Valium) *Phenothiazines* Promethazine hydrochloride (Phenergan), propiomazine hydrochloride (Largon), hydroxyzine pamoate (Vistaril), promazine hydrochloride (Sparine) *Parasympatholytics* Atropine *General anesthetics*	
3. Fetal sleep cycles Periods of fetal sleep, usually lasting for 20 to 30 minutes, produce decreased LTV; does not usually affect STV	Variability that is decreased as a result of fetal sleep patterns usually resumes in 20 to 30 minutes
4. Congenital anomalies Central nervous system (e.g., anencephaly) or cardiac anomalies can decrease variability	No intervention can reverse congenital anomalies
5. Fetal cardiac arrhythmias Suppression of cardiac control mechanisms may be the result of paroxysmal atrial tachycardia, complete heart block, nodal rhythm, or an aberrant pacemaker	Some cardiac drugs may be given via the mother in an attempt to cardiovert some arrhythmias

Cause of Variations in Variability	Clinical Significance/Intervention
6. Extreme prematurity (<24 weeks) Heartbeat is controlled by immature neurological mechanisms, resulting in even intervals from one heartbeat to the next	No intervention can reverse extreme prematurity

Intervention
Increased baseline variability

Observe the FHR tracing carefully for any sign of fetal distress, including periodic changes and increases or decreases in baseline FHR. Consider using the internal spiral electrode if the pattern is observed during external monitoring, especially if there is a concern of change in fetal condition and a decreased tolerance of labor.

Decreased baseline variability

Intervention is dependent on the cause. Intervention is not warranted if decreased variability is associated with fetal sleep cycles or if it is temporarily associated with prescribed CNS depressants. Application of the spiral electrode should be considered if the pattern is observed using external monitoring and the quality of the tracing is not consistently interpretable. If a central nervous system–depressant drug has been given near the time of delivery, Narcan is routinely administered to the neonate after delivery. If hypoxia is suspected, turning the patient on her side and administering oxygen may improve oxygen saturation. Monitoring fetal oxygen saturation ($FSpO_2$) may provide additional clinical information. In addition, hydration and elimination of uterine hyperstimulation may enhance fetal oxygenation and uteroplacental blood flow.

Tachycardia
Definition

Fetal tachycardia is defined as a baseline heart rate ≥ 160 bpm for a duration of 10 minutes or more (NICHD, 1997; Parer, 1997; Freeman, Garite, Nageotte, 1991).

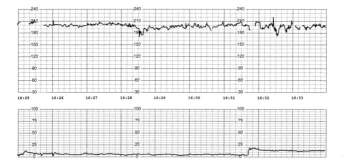

Figure 5-5
Fetal tachycardia.

Description

Fetal tachycardia is usually secondary to maternal fever, beta-sympathomimetic drugs, amnionitis, congenital infection, or hyper-thyroidism. However, a fetus that is less than 32 weeks' gestation may have a FHR around 160 bpm. As gestational age increases, baseline FHR gradually decreases. Tachycardia is the result of an increase in sympathetic and decrease in parasympathetic tone and is sometimes associated with a decrease or loss of FHR variability. Tachycardia may be a sign of early fetal hypoxia when associated with periodic changes and decreasing baseline variability. Therefore it is important to assess the FHR for increases in baseline rate, a decrease in variability, periodic changes, and the duration of the patterns observed (Figure 5-5).

Causes

Causes	Mechanism
1. Fetal hypoxia	1. Fetus attempts to compensate for reduced blood flow by increase of sympathetic stimulation or release of epinephrine from adrenal medulla, or both

Causes	Mechanism
2. Maternal fever	2. Accelerates metabolism of fetal myocardium; increases sympathetic cardioacceleration activity up to 2 hours before the mother is febrile
3. Parasympatholytic drugs (e.g., atropine, scopolamine, hydroxyzine [Vistaril, Atarax], phenothiazines)	3. Block the parasympathetic pathway of the autonomic nervous system
4. Beta-sympathomimetic drugs (e.g., terbutaline and ritodrine)	4. These tocolytic drugs, given to control labor, have a cardiac stimulant effect similar to that of epinephrine
5. Illicit drugs (e.g., cocaine and methamphetamines)	5. Epinephrine/norepinephrine response that causes increased maternal and fetal heart rate
6. Amnionitis	6. Increased heart rate can be the first sign of developing intrauterine infection (as with prolonged rupture of membranes)
7. Maternal hyperthyroidism	7. Long-acting thyroid-stimulating hormones (LATS) probably cross the placenta and increase FHR
8. Fetal anemia	8. FHR increases in an effort to increase cardiac output and tissue perfusion
9. Fetal heart failure	9. The fetal heart attempts to compensate for failure by concurrently increasing rate and cardiac output; can occur as a result of tachyarrhythmia

Causes	Mechanism
10. Fetal cardiac arrhythmias*	10. Tachyarrhythmias and variations of normal sinus rhythm may occur (e.g., paroxysmal atrial tachycardia [PAT], atrial flutter, and premature ventricular contractions [PVCs]); congenital cardiac anomaly may be present; FHR in excess of 240 bpm cannot be followed by monitor because this exceeds FHR range parameters or the rate may be halved because of limitations of the monitor

Clinical Significance

Three types of fetal tachycardia are sinus tachycardia, atrial flutter/fibrillation, and supraventricular tachycardia. Sinus tachycardia, with a rate above 160 bpm, may be the result of a drug effect or a response to maternal infection such as amnionitis. It is not necessarily a sign of fetal hypoxia unless it is associated with repetitive late decelerations and/or lack of variability. Atrial flutter/fibrillation, with an atrial rate between 300 and 450 bpm, is rarely diagnosed in the antepartum period and is associated with a high mortality rate.

Supraventricular tachycardia (SVT), with a heart rate in excess of 200 bpm, is the most frequently occurring form of fetal tachyarrhythmia. Short periods of SVT are of no clinical significance. However, longer periods of SVT have been associated with high cardiac output failure, nonimmune hydrops fetalis, ascites, hydramnios, and fetal death.

Tachycardia can be a nonreassuring sign when associated with late decelerations or absence of variability. In terms of immediate neonatal outcome, persistent tachycardia with moderate (average) baseline variability or in the absence of periodic changes (e.g., decelerations) does not appear to adversely compromise the fetus and is rarely associated with fetal asphyxia. This is particularly true when tachycardia is associated with maternal fever.

Fetal cardiac arrhythmias may be confused with electrical noise or maternal ECG artifact on the fetal monitor because they are characterized by large vertical excursions on the FHR scale. They can, however, be diagnosed through the use of spiral electrode, real-time ultrasound, and turning off the logic switch and checking the electronic fetal monitor for malfunction.

Intervention

Intervention for tachycardia is dependent on etiological factors. Maternal fever can be reduced with antipyretics and hydration. If maternal oxygenation is an issue, 100% oxygen at 8 to 10 L/min via snug face mask may improve or optimize fetal oxygenation by supersaturating maternal plasma oxygen levels. When the diagnosis of SVT is made, in utero therapy of the premature fetus or delivery of the mature fetus must be initiated. In utero treatment can consist of maternal administration of a single drug or combinations of digoxin, calcium channel blockers (nifedipine), beta-blockers (propranolol [Inderal]), and antiarrhythmic agents such as procainamide and quinidine, which crosses the placental barrier and treats the fetus.

Bradycardia

Definition

Fetal bradycardia is defined as a baseline heart rate ≤ 110 bpm for a duration of 10 minutes or more (NICHD, 1997; Parer, 1997; Freeman, Garite, Nageotte, 1991).

Description

Bradycardia is frequently the response of the fetus to hypoxia; however, there are nonasphyxial causes of bradycardia, including heart block and congenital cardiac anomalies. Bradycardia with good variability may be associated with occiput posterior or transverse position and is probably the result of increased vagal tone (Freeman, Garite, Nageotte, 1991). When bradycardia is detected at the initiation of monitoring it is difficult to distinguish it from a prolonged deceleration. Bradycardia is generally a late sign of fetal hypoxia indicative of progressive acidosis when associated with periodic changes and decreasing baseline variability. Therefore it is important to assess the FHR for a decrease in baseline rate, a decrease in variability, periodic changes, and the duration of the patterns observed (Figure 5-6).

Causes

Causes	Mechanism
1. Late (profound) fetal hypoxia	1. Myocardial activity becomes depressed and lowers heart rate

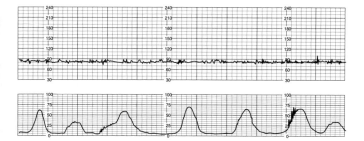

Figure 5-6
Fetal bradycardia.

Causes	Mechanism
2. Beta-adrenergic blocking drugs (e.g., propranolol)	2. Epinephrine receptor sites in the myocardium are blocked by these drugs, permitting unopposed vagal tone and a decreased heart rate
3. Anesthetics (epidural, spinal, and pudendal)	3. Bradycardia may develop indirectly because of a reflex mechanism or because of maternal hypotension produced by maternal supine position, insufficient preanesthesia hydration, or the sympathetic blockade response to the anesthetic agent
4. Maternal hypotension	4. Maternal supine position causes uterine compression of the vena cava, which results in hypotension syndrome (a decrease in maternal cardiac output and blood pressure, which decreases uteroplacental blood flow, resulting in a subsequent decrease in FHR)
5. Prolonged umbilical cord compression	5. Cord compression triggers sensitization of fetal baroceptors, resulting in vagal stimulation and decreased heart rate
6. Fetal cardiac arrhythmias	6. FHR can be low (70 to 90 bpm) with bradyarrhythmias (complete heart block)

Causes	Mechanism
7. Hypothermia	7. Maternal (and therefore fetal) hypothermia reduces myocardial metabolism, decreases oxygen requirements, and decreases heart rate
8. Maternal systemic lupus erythematosus	8. Complete atrioventricular dissociation associated with connective tissue disease produces persistent bradycardia
9. Cytomegalovirus (CMV)	9. Structural cardiac defects may occur with CMV infection, resulting in congenital heart block expressed as fetal bradycardia
10. Prolonged maternal hypoglycemia	10. Maternal and subsequently fetal hypoglycemia can potentiate hypoxemia with a depression of myocardial activity and decreased heart rate
11. Congenital heart block	11. Congenital heart block of first, second, or third degree can result in bradycardia. First-degree block does not require treatment in the fetus and has not yet been reported in the literature. In second-degree block not all the impulses from the sinoatrial node in the atria are conducted to the ventricles. Mobitz type I block is evidenced by a progressive lengthening of the PR interval and is rarely of any significance. Mobitz type II block occurs infrequently but is more serious and often a precursor to third-degree, or complete, heart block. Complete heart block is most often associated with congenital heart disease.

Clinical Significance

Bradycardia resulting from hypoxia is a nonreassuring sign when associated with loss of variability and late decelerations. Substantial bradycardia with absent baseline variability, especially when prolonged and uncorrectable, is predictive of current or impending fetal asphyxia of such severity that the fetus is at risk of neurological and other fetal damage or death (NICHD, 1997). Bradycardia in the 100- to 110-bpm range with average FHR variability and absence of late decelerations is not usually a sign of fetal distress. Intervention is also not warranted in fetuses with heart block diagnosed in the antepartum period.

Although paracervical blocks are rarely performed, the resultant bradycardia is usually transitory with recovery occurring in utero. The 5-minute Apgar is usually above 7 if the FHR pattern was reassuring before the onset of the bradycardia and if delivery does not occur during the paracervical block bradycardia. Poor fetal outcome has occurred with delivery during the resulting bradycardia caused by fetal hypoxia and acidosis. Neonatal resuscitation and stabilization is indicated until the paracervical pharmacological agent has been metabolized.

Intervention

Intervention for bradycardia is dependent on etiological factors. Clinical judgment and resulting intervention are based on a variety of factors, including stage of labor, presentation and station of fetus, and indications of fetal stress. Maternal positioning (lateral), hydration, correction of maternal hypotension, maternal oxygenation at 8 to 10 L/min at 100% by snug face mask, and elimination of uterine hyperstimulation are indicated to optimize and improve fetal oxygenation. In addition, scalp stimulation can be performed in an effort to produce FHR acceleration in order to establish whether the fetus has the ability to mobilize oxygen and physiologically compensate for stress. In addition, monitoring fetal oxygen saturation ($FSpO_2$) may provide additional clinical information. Infants delivered with congenital heart block may require a pacemaker.

Unusual Patterns
Sinusoidal Pattern

A sinusoidal FHR pattern (Figure 5-7) is a *sine* wave characterized by an *undulating* baseline and the following features:
1. Regular oscillations with an amplitude range of up to 30 bpm
2. Frequency of 2 to 6 cycles/min of long-term variability
3. Minimal to absent short-term variability
4. Rhythmic oscillation of a sine wave above and below a baseline
5. Absence of FHR accelerations in response to fetal movement
6. Extreme regularity and smoothness

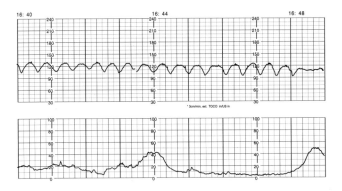

Figure 5-7
Sinusoidal FHR.

This pattern has been known to occur in the presence of fetal hypoxia, often as a result of Rh isoimmunization, fetal anemia, and chronic fetal bleeds. In these cases it has been associated with an increase in fetal morbidity and mortality, and survival may depend on extrauterine support in a neonatal intensive care unit.

The pattern has also been reported after the administration of analgesics, such as alphaprodine (Nisentil), meperidine (Demerol), and butorphanol tartrate (Stadol), and in association with amnionitis. The pattern following the administration of these drugs is termed *pseudosinusoidal* and is usually a temporary phenomenon not associated with an adverse fetal outcome; the pattern may be corrected after a dose of Narcan. Pseudosinusoidal patterns are characterized by sine waves that are less uniform, and STV is usually present. In addition, these patterns are preceded and followed by normal FHR patterns.

If there is a persistent, uncorrectable sinusoidal pattern and other signs of fetal compromise are present, expeditious delivery may be indicated. If the pattern is inconsistent and apparently transitory after intravenous narcotics, fetal compromise is not expected.

Fetal Cardiac Arrhythmias

Fetal cardiac arrhythmias occur in many pregnancies. Tachycardia and bradycardia have been previously discussed in this chapter. Other arrhythmias include:

1. Premature atrial contractions (PACs) and premature ventricular contractions (PVCs)

    1. These are represented on the tracing as vertical excursions above or below the FHR baseline. PACs and PVCs usually have no clinical significance and do not require intervention.

2. Transient fetal cardiac asystole

    2. Transient fetal cardiac asystole may be evidenced by a rapid downward deflection of the FHR followed quickly by a rapid upward excursion back to the previous FHR baseline. This has been reported during the nadir of severe variable decelerations. Management should include position change, vaginal examination to rule out cord prolapse or rapid fetal descent, and elevation of the presenting part as indicated.

It is important to distinguish fetal arrhythmias from electrical noise or maternal ECG artifact, because they can all be evidenced by the same pattern. To adequately discriminate fetal arrhythmias from noise and artifact, diagnoses can be achieved by spiral electrode, real-time ultrasound, turning off the logic switch, and checking the electronic fetal monitor for malfunction.

Isolated extrasystoles, most of which are supraventricular in orgin, are of little clinical importance and are the major disturbance of fetal cardiac rhythm. On auscultation this sounds like a skipped beat, but it is usually either a pause after an extrasystole or an undetectable heartbeat. There are, however, other tachyarrhythmias and bradyarrhythmias of supraventricular or ventricular origin that can be evaluated with M-mode, pulsed Doppler, or color-encoded fetal echocardiography. The majority of fetal cardiac arrhythmias resolve spontaneously in late pregnancy or during the first few days after birth. The treatment of arrhythmias is one of the most specialized disciplines of cardiology and not without significant potential risk of undesired effects. The use of antiarrhythmic drugs must be based on a thorough understanding of the electrophysiology of the arrhythmia, as well as the electrophysiological and hemodynamic effects of the chemotherapeutic agents. The interactive potential between potent antiarrhythmic agents must be considered as well. The action of these drugs alters the electrophysiological activity of the heart by altering ion flux at the level of ion channels within the cell membrane. Drug interactions at the cellular level have the potential for impairing myocardial performance and interfering with metabolism of other drugs and could result in a proarrhythmic effect, that is, to cause rather than ameliorate an arrhythmia.

On occasion, antiarrhythmic therapy is initiated in specialized tertiary centers on an inpatient basis after risk/benefit analysis and consultation with the obstetrician, pediatric cardiologist, and informed parents. The fetus is continually monitored before, during, and after administration of the antiarrhythmic agent to the mother, who is continually monitored with a 12-lead ECG, as well as baseline and ongoing maternal blood studies (Kleinman, Nehgme, Copel, 1999).

Summary of Baseline Changes

	Tachycardia
Definition	Sustained FHR above 160 bpm for more than 10 minutes
Etiology	Early fetal hypoxia, drugs, maternal fever, amnionitis, fetal anemia, fetal heart failure, and/or cardiac arrhythmias
Clinical significance	Usually benign when associated with maternal fever
	Nonreassuring when associated with late decelerations, loss of variability, or severe variable decelerations
Nursing intervention	Dependent on etiological factors; reduce maternal fever with hydration and antipyretics; lateral position change and oxygen at 8 to 10 L/min by snug face mask
	For supraventricular tachycardia, in utero treatment can consist of maternal administration of a single drug or combinations of digoxin, calcium channel blockers (nifedipine), beta-blockers (propranolol [Inderal]), and antiarrhythmic agents such as procainamide and quinidine, which cross the placental barrier and treat the fetus

Bradycardia	Minimal to Absent Variability
Sustained FHR below 110 bpm for more than 10 minutes	*Baseline variability:* Rhythmic fluctuations in the baseline FHR of 2 cycles per minute or greater; irregular in amplitude and frequency
	Short term: changes in FHR from one beat to the next
Late (profound) fetal hypoxia, drugs, maternal hypotension, prolapsed cord, or congenital heart block	*Decreased variability:* Prematurity, drugs, hypoxia, fetal sleep, congenital anomalies, fetal cardiac arrhythmias, central nervous system depression
Bradycardia of 100 to 110 bpm without periodic deceleration and with average FHR variability is not usually a sign of fetal hypoxia	Benign when associated with periodic fetal sleep; return of variability usually occurs when drugs are excreted or metabolized
Nonreassuring when associated with late decelerations or loss of variability; indicates profound fetal distress	Ominous when associated with late decelerations and severe variable decelerations
Dependent on etiological factors; lateral position change and oxygen at 8 to 10 L/min by snug face mask may be of some value; eliminate uterine hyperstimulation to improve fetal oxygenation and uteroplacental blood flow; scalp stimulation can be performed in an effort to produce FHR acceleration to demonstrate physiologic compensation for stress; $FSpO_2$ may provide additional clinical information. Intervention is not warranted in fetus with heart block diagnosed by ECG in the antepartum period	Dependent on etiological factors; fetal oxygen saturation ($FSpO_2$) monitoring may provide additional clinical information; intervention is not warranted if associated with fetal sleep cycle or temporarily associated with central nervous system depressants

Periodic and Nonperiodic Changes

6

Periodic changes in fetal heart rate (FHR) are transient accelerations or decelerations from the baseline, after which the FHR returns to baseline. These changes occur in response to uterine contractions and may begin as compensatory mechanisms or precursors to hypoxia.

Nonperiodic or *episodic changes* are accelerations or decelerations that occur without any specific relationship to uterine activity. They can include spontaneous accelerations and variable decelerations between contractions and prolonged decelerations.

All FHR changes, whether periodic or nonperiodic, should be systematically evaluated within the parameters of the "company they keep" (Chez, 1992). These parameters include FHR baseline and variability before, during, and after the change; presence of combined changes (e.g., lates and variables); change related to uterine activity or resting tone (e.g., hyperstimulation and increased resting tone); and general information that is available about maternal and fetal condition. By doing this complete assessment, the clinician remains aware of changes that suggest levels of hypoxia (mild to worsening), as well as the presence or absence of compensatory mechanisms that give an indication of the level of oxygen reserve in fetal tissue. Further assessment can be achieved by monitoring fetal oxygen saturation ($FSpO_2$) to provide additional clinical information. Timely and appropriate interventions then follow the evaluation of the FHR pattern and determination of fetal tolerance to labor.

Accelerations
Definition

Acceleration is defined as a visually apparent abrupt increase in FHR above the baseline. The onset of the acceleration to its peak is less than 30 seconds. The increase is calculated from the most recently determined portion of the baseline. The acme is more than 15 bpm above the baseline, and the acceleration lasts more than 15 seconds but less than 2 minutes from the onset of the acceleration to the return to baseline. Before 32 weeks' gestation, accelerations are defined as having an acme of more than 10 bpm above the baseline for a duration of more than 10 seconds.

A prolonged acceleration is of a duration of 2 minutes or more but less than 10 minutes. An apparent acceleration that lasts 10 minutes or more is a change of FHR baseline (NICHD, 1997).

Description

The majority of accelerations of FHR from the baseline are episodic and not associated with uterine contractions (UC). These nonperiodic accelerations are most often associated with fetal movement, stimulation, or environmental stimuli. Accelerations of FHR with fetal movement are considered reassuring and form the basis for the Non-Stress Test (NST).

When accelerations are associated with uterine contractions they are considered to be a periodic change. Repetitive accelerations with uterine contractions are observed less frequently than spontaneous episodic accelerations.

Characteristics

	Episodic/Spontaneous (Not Associated With UC)	Periodic (Associated With UC)
SHAPE	Transitory increase in baseline	Resembles shape of UC; may be biphasic or triphasic
ONSET	Can occur at any time; onset to peak <30 seconds	Before or after peak of UC; onset to peak <30 seconds
RECOVERY	Variable; >15 seconds to <2 minutes from onset of acceleration to return to baseline	Return to baseline can occur after or at the same time as the uterine pressure returns to its resting tone; ≥15 seconds to <2 minutes from onset

	Episodic/Spontaneous (Not Associated With UC)	Periodic (Associated With UC)
		of acceleration to return to baseline
ACCELERATION	Usually ≥15 bpm above baseline for ≥15 seconds; if fetus <32 weeks' gestation, acme is ≥10 bpm above baseline with duration of ≥10 seconds	Usually ≥15 bpm above baseline for ≥15 seconds; if fetus <32 weeks' gestation, acme is ≥10 bpm above baseline with duration of ≥10 seconds
BASELINE	Associated with average baseline variability	Sometimes associated with decreasing or smooth baseline variability
OCCURRENCE	Variable; can occur at any time; usually in response to fetal movement or stimulation	Repetitious; tends to occur with each contraction

Etiology

Stimulation of the sympathetic division of the autonomic nervous system can accelerate the fetal heart rate. FHR accelerations can be associated with the following:

1. Spontaneous fetal movement
2. Vaginal examination
3. Application of the spiral electrode
4. Breech presentation
5. Occiput posterior presentation
6. Uterine contractions
7. Fundal pressure
8. Abdominal palpation
9. Vibroacoustic stimulation
10. Scalp stimulation
11. Environmental stimuli (e.g., noise)

Clinical Significance

Episodic or spontaneous (nonperiodic) accelerations of FHR in response to fetal movement and fetal stimulation are associated with an intact fetal central nervous system and fetal well-being. Accelerations of FHR in the intrapartum period associated with fetal movement and fetal stimulation are reassuring. Fetal movement can be identified on the uterine activity (UA) panel as spikes or momentary increases in uterine pressure on the lower section of the monitor strip. Accelerations may be seen in response to stimulation of the fetal head as occurs with vaginal examinations and insertion of a scalp electrode or intrauterine pressure catheter (IUPC).

Periodic repetitive accelerations that are associated with uterine contractions may be the earliest indicator of possible partial cord compression. This can be secondary to baroreceptor-induced transient increase in FHR that occurs as a result of fetal hypotension produced when a uterine contraction compresses the umbilical cord. This compensatory mechanism reflects a healthy fetus with an appropriate cardiovascular response (Figure 6-1).

Intervention

Acceleration of FHR is considered a benign pattern, and no intervention is required. If partial cord compression is suspected, maternal repositioning should be done. However, it would be wise to observe repetitive accelerations in association with uterine

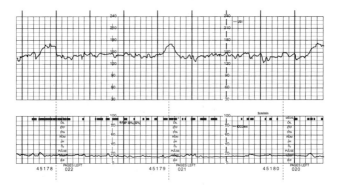

Figure 6-1
Acceleration of FHR with fetal movement.

contractions in the event they evolve into FHR decelerations as labor progresses.

Early Decelerations

Definition

Early deceleration of the fetal heart rate is a periodic change that is associated with a uterine contraction. It is a visually apparent gradual decrease (defined as onset of deceleration to nadir in 30 seconds or more) and return to the baseline FHR. The decrease is determined from the most recently determined portion of the baseline. It is coincident in timing, with the nadir of the deceleration occurring at the same time as the peak of the uterine contraction (NICHD, 1997).

Description

Early decelerations are caused by head compression. They begin early in the contracting phase, with the onset usually before the peak of the uterine contraction and the recovery occurring at the same time the uterine contraction returns to the baseline. The timing is synchronous with that of the contraction. Generally this pattern occurs more frequently during the active phase of labor, initially occurring between 4 and 7 cm of dilatation, primarily in primagravidas, but may be present until cervical dilatation is complete at 10 cm. Early decelerations are benign changes that occur as a result of compression of the fetal head (ACOG, 1995d; Freeman, Garite, Nageotte, 1991).

Physiology

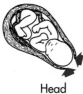

Head
compression

Pressure on the fetal skull
↓
Alters cerebral blood flow
↓
Stimulates central vagus nerve
↓
Produces decrease in heart rate with
↓
Recovery occurring as pressure
is relieved

Characteristics (Figure 6-2)

SHAPE	Uniform shape; a "mirror image" of the contraction phase
ONSET	Early in the contraction phase; before the peak of the contraction; onset to nadir ≥30 seconds; nadir, or low point, of the deceleration occurs at the same time as the peak of the contraction
RECOVERY	Return to baseline occurs by the end of the contraction as uterine pressure returns to its resting tone
DECELERATION	Rarely decelerates below 110 bpm, or 20 to 30 bpm below baseline; amplitude of deceleration is usually proportional to amplitude of contraction
BASELINE	Usually associated with average baseline variability
OCCURRENCE	Repetitious; occurs with each contraction; usually observed between 4 and 7 cm dilatation; observed when there is head compression

Etiology

This pattern is a result of direct vagal stimulation of the temporal baroreceptors as a result of descent and increased pressure on the head as it passes through the pelvic outlet and vaginal canal. Head compression decelerations can result from the following:

1. Uterine contractions
2. Cephalopelvic disproportion
3. Persistent occiput posterior

Clinical Significance

Early decelerations, caused by head compression, have no pathological significance. They do not occur in all labors, but when they do appear they are repetitive and associated with uterine contractions. They are not associated with decreasing baseline variability nor changes in baseline FHR.

A *transient deceleration* of FHR may occur with vaginal examinations, placement of the internal scalp electrode or intrauterine pressure catheter, or fundal pressure. These should not be

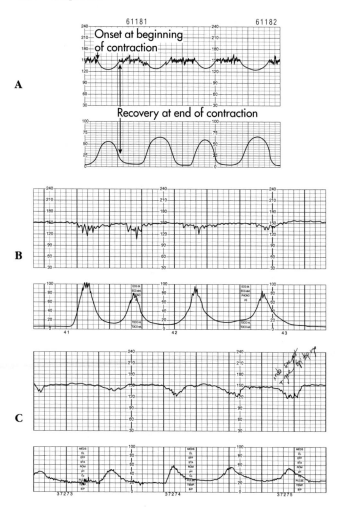

Figure 6-2
A, Early decelerations (illustration with key points identified). **B** and **C,** Early decelerations (actual tracings).

confused with early decelerations that are a periodic change, repetitive, and associated with uterine contractions.

Intervention

Early decelerations are a benign pattern, and no intervention is required. The importance of identifying early decelerations is to be able to distinguish them from late and variable decelerations.

Late Decelerations

Definition

Late deceleration of the fetal heart rate is a visually apparent gradual decrease and return to baseline FHR associated with a uterine contraction. The timing of the onset to nadir is 30 seconds or more. The decrease is determined from the most recently determined portion of the baseline. The deceleration is delayed in time, with the nadir of the deceleration occurring after the peak of the contraction (NICHD, 1997).

Description

Late decelerations are those that begin late in the contracting phase. The onset of the deceleration occurs after the onset of the uterine contraction, with the depth of the nadir occurring after the peak or acme of the contraction. The recovery of the deceleration usually occurs after the return of the contraction to the uterine activity baseline. Late decelerations are repetitive periodic changes (associated with uterine contractions), indicative of uteroplacental insufficiency, and are nonreassuring.

Physiology

Uteroplacental
insufficiency

Uterine hyperactivity
or maternal hypo-
tension

↓

Decreases intervillous
space blood flow
during uterine
contractions

↓

Decreases maternal/fetal oxygen transfer

↓

Produces fetal hypoxia
and myocardial
depression

↓

Activates vagal
response

↓

Produces cardio-
deceleration   ←   Lactic acidosis

True placental
dysfunction

↓

Anaerobic
metabolism

Characteristics (Figure 6-3)

SHAPE	Uniform shape; a "mirror image" of the contraction phase, deep or shallow depending upon the degree of hypoxia
ONSET	Late in the contraction phase; onset to nadir ≥30 seconds; nadir, or low point, of the deceleration occurs after the peak of the contraction
RECOVERY	Return to the baseline occurs after the end of the contraction (usually >20 seconds after uterine pressure returns to its resting tone)
DECELERATION	Rarely decelerates below 100 bpm; amplitude of deceleration is usually proportional to amplitude of contraction; *persistent, uncorrected* decelerations of *any* magnitude are nonreassuring, and the most depressed

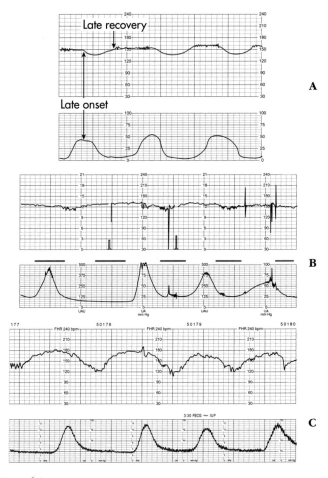

Figure 6-3
A, Late decelerations (illustration with key points identified).
B and **C,** Late decelerations (actual tracings).

	fetuses may have only shallow or subtle late decelerations (e.g., 3 to 5 bpm)
BASELINE	Often associated with loss of variability and a rising baseline or tachycardia; variability may be increased or decreased during the nadir of the deceleration
OCCURRENCE	Repetitious; occurs with each contraction; can be observed at any time during labor when there is uteroplacental insufficiency

Etiology

Uteroplacental insufficiency can result from the following:

Cause	Mechanism
1. Hyperstimulation of the uterus from oxytocin augmentation or induction	1. Hyperstimulation enhances vasoconstriction, reduces cardiac output, and decreases intervillous space blood flow
2. Maternal spine hypotension	2. Compression of the inferior vena cava reduces venous return and maternal cardiac output
3. Pregnancy-induced hypertension	3. Vasospasm occurring in uterine vessels decreases intervillous space blood flow and produces fetal hypoxia
4. Chronic hypertension	4. Hypertensive vascular disease constricts blood vessels and reduces intervillous blood flow, thus producing fetal hypoxia
5. Postmaturity	5. Fetus "outgrows" placenta; insufficient function of the placenta reduces supply of oxygen and nutrients to the fetus

Cause	Mechanism
6. Amnionitis	6. Maternal infection reduces the efficiency of the utero-placental unit; related fetal tachycardia increases the metabolic rate, rapidly depleting placental oxygen reserves; amnionitis often causes uterine hyperactivity, which decreases intervillous space blood flow and leads to fetal hypoxia
7. Small for gestational age (SGA)	7. Intrauterine growth restriction (IUGR) with reduced fetal placental reserve
8. Maternal diabetes	8. Maternal vascular involvement and sclerotic arterial changes reduce uteroplacental perfusion
9. Placenta previa	9. Placental attachment to the lower uterine segment (covering internal cervical os) may cause early separation and increase chance of hemorrhage
10. Abruptio placentae/maternal shock	10. Premature separation of placenta decreases functioning placental area and related uterine hyperactivity
11. Regional anesthetics (spinal, epidural)	11. May cause maternal hypotension, reducing blood flow to uteroplacental unit
12. Maternal cardiac disease	12. Conditions that affect pumping of blood reduce blood flow to uteroplacental unit; cyanotic conditions reduce oxygen content of blood flowing to placenta
13. Maternal anemia	13. Reduction of RBCs or hemoglobin decreases the

Cause	Mechanism
	amount of oxygen to feto-placental unit
14. Rh isoimmunization	14. Fetal anemia decreases the amount of available oxygen, and the hypoxic stress occurring with a uterine contraction can precipitate metabolic acidosis
15. Other conditions: collagen vascular disease, renal disease, and advanced maternal age	15. Conditions compromise placental exchange because of sclerotic arterial and venous changes

Clinical Significance

Late decelerations of any magnitude should be considered a non-reassuring sign when they are persistent and uncorrectable, especially when associated with tachycardia and/or minimal or absent variability. As myocardial depression increases, the depth of the late deceleration decreases, becoming more subtle or shallow in appearance. In contrast, a single late deceleration in an otherwise reassuring pattern is not clinically significant.

Persistent and uncorrectable late decelerations reflect repetitive hypoxic stress and if associated with minimal or absent variability become a sign of increasing metabolic acidosis.

Intervention

Procedure*	Rationale
1. Change maternal position to lateral	1. Decreases pressure on the inferior vena cava and corrects supine hypotension
2. Correct maternal hypotension a. Lower head	2. a. Increases venous return and promotes cardiac output

*Consider placement of internal electrode as appropriate for better assessment of FHR.

Procedure	Rationale
b. Increase rate of mainte-nance IV infusion	b. Increases maternal circu-lating volume and cardiac output; this can facilitate excretion of oxytocin
c. Administer vasopressors (e.g., ephedrine sulfate) for severe unresponsive hypotension caused by conduction anesthesia	c. Increases blood pressure by increasing arteriolar constriction and cardiac stimulation
3. Discontinue oxytocin if infus-ing	3. Decreases uterine activity
4. Administer oxygen 8 to 10 L/min at 100% by snug face mask	4. Increases fetal oxygen satura-tion ($FSpO_2$) of hemoglobin with maximum increase after about 9 minutes of 100% O_2 to the mother (McNamara, Johnson, Lilford, 1993)
5. Fetal scalp or acoustic stimu-lation	5. May be useful to elicit an acceleration of FHR that would not be indicative of fetal acidosis
6. Fetal oxygen saturation ($FSpO_2$) monitoring may be considered	6. To distinguish normoxia from hypoxia in the fetus; values less than 30% indicates aci-dosis
7. Termination of labor is con-sidered by the physician if the pattern cannot be cor-rected, particularly if vari-ability is decreasing and an acceleration of FHR cannot be elicited	7. Continuation of labor can only further compromise the fetus by increasing hypoxia and acidosis

Variable Decelerations
Definition

Variable deceleration of the fetal heart rate is defined as a visually apparent *abrupt* decrease in FHR below the baseline. The onset of the deceleration to the beginning of the nadir is less than 30 seconds. The decrease is determined from the most recently determined portion of the baseline. The decrease in FHR below the baseline is 15 or more beats per minute, lasting 15 or more seconds but less than 2 minutes from onset to return to baseline (NICHD, 1997).

Description

Variable decelerations are episodic changes caused by umbilical cord compression. They can occur with any interruption in umbilical blood flow at any time during labor but are often concurrent with uterine contractions. The decelerations vary in the depth of the nadir, and duration is less than 2 minutes. They frequently decelerate below the average FHR range. Variable decelerations are the most frequently observed FHR pattern in labor.

Physiology

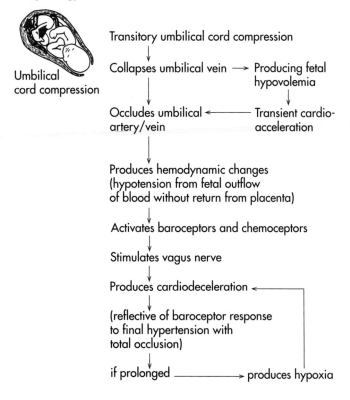

Umbilical
cord compression

Transitory umbilical cord compression
↓
Collapses umbilical vein ⟶ Producing fetal
hypovolemia
↓
Occludes umbilical ⟵ Transient cardio-
artery/vein   acceleration
↓
Produces hemodynamic changes
(hypotension from fetal outflow
of blood without return from placenta)
↓
Activates baroceptors and chemoceptors
↓
Stimulates vagus nerve
↓
Produces cardiodeceleration ⟵
↓
(reflective of baroceptor response
to final hypertension with
total occlusion)
↓
if prolonged ⟶ produces hypoxia

Characteristics

SHAPE	Variable; does not reflect the shape of any associated uterine contraction; characterized by an abrupt drop in heart rate in a ᐯ "V," or ᐁ "U," or "W" shape
ONSET	Variable times in the contraction phase; onset to beginning of nadir <30 seconds; often preceded and followed by transitory acceleration (shouldering)
RECOVERY	Return to baseline occurs rapidly, sometimes with transitory acceleration (shouldering), ᐯ, or ᐯ overshoot
DECELERATION	FHR decrease is ≥15 bpm; often decelerates below 100 bpm; lasts ≥15 seconds but <2 minutes
BASELINE	May be associated with average baseline variability or decreased variability with significant hypoxia
OCCURRENCE	Observed when there is cord compression; not necessarily repetitive; frequently observed late in labor; may be associated with pushing in the second stage of labor

Variations (Figures 6-4 to 6-6)

Variable decelerations have been graded based on the depth of the nadir and the duration of the decelerations; however, these are rough quantitative estimations of the severity of variable decelerations (Kubli et al, 1969). This grading does not consider other parameters such as an increase/decrease in baseline rate nor diminishing or absent variability. In order to fully evaluate the severity of variable decelerations, the baseline rate and variability must be evaluated. This grading is meant to be useful in assessing the monitor strip for any progression in the duration and nadir of variable decelerations.

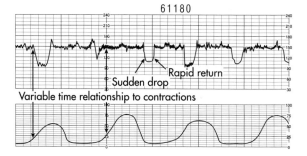

Figure 6-4
Mild variable decelerations (illustration with key points identified).

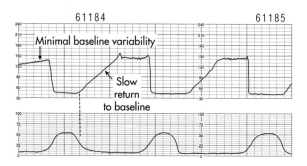

Figure 6-5
Severe variable decelerations (illustration with key points identified).

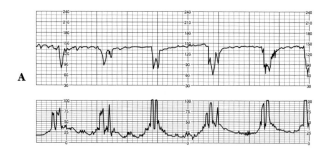

Figure 6-6
A-D, Variable decelerations. Note the progression in severity from Panel *A* to *E* with overshoots and decreasing variability and eventual prolonged deceleration (actual tracings).

Continued

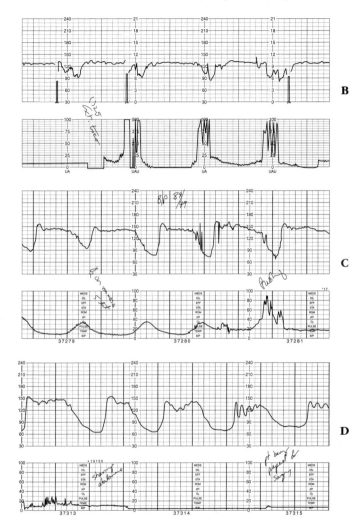

B

C

D

Figure 6-6
For legend, see opposite page.   *Continued*

E

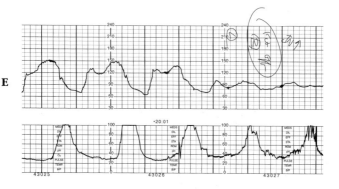

Figure 6-6, cont'd
For legend see p. 112.

Grading based on duration of nadir of variable decelerations follows:

Mild	Moderate	Severe
Any level for <30 seconds *or* 70 to 80 bpm for <60 seconds *or* >80 bpm for any duration	<70 bpm for 30 to 60 seconds *or* 70 to 80 bpm for >60 seconds	<70 bpm for >60 seconds

Etiology

Interruption in umbilical blood flow can result from the following:
1. Maternal position; cord between fetus and maternal pelvis
2. Cord around fetal neck (nuchal cord), leg, arm, or other body part
3. Short cord
4. Knot in cord
5. Prolapsed cord
6. Fetal movement in presence of oligohydramnios

Clinical Significance

Variable decelerations indicate umbilical cord compression. They occur in about 50% of all labors and are usually transient and correctable phenomena. They vary in duration, depth (nadir), and timing relative to uterine contraction and any other type of interruption in umbilical blood flow. When variable decelerations are associated with uterine contractions, their onset, depth, and duration commonly vary with successive uterine contractions (NICHD, 1997).

Progression of variable decelerations are more important than absolute parameters in distinguishing those that are reassuring from those that are nonreassurring (ACOG, 1995d). For example, a *mild variable deceleration* is considered to be one that decelerates to any level for less than 30 seconds because it is very abrupt in both onset and return to baseline. This is considered a reassuring variable deceleration. When variable decelerations become persistent, progressively deeper, and longer lasting with a prolonged return to baseline they are considered nonreassuring. For example, a *severe variable deceleration* is below 70 bpm for longer than 60 seconds with a slow return to baseline. The progressively prolonged return to baseline is of concern because it reflects the development and progression of hypoxia (Freeman, Garite, Nageotte, 1991). Severe variable decelerations may also be accompanied by an increase in baseline rate with a decrease in baseline variability.

Shouldering or overshoot may occur with variable decelerations. *Shouldering* is a transient preacceleratory and postacceleratory phase of the FHR, generally lasting less than 20 seconds at the beginning and end of the deceleration. These increases in FHR above the baseline before and after the variable deceleration has reached its nadir appear to "shoulder" the deceleration. This is considered to be a normal physiological compensatory mechanism. *Overshoot* is a transitory acceleration of the FHR that occurs at the end of a variable deceleration. After the variable deceleration has reached its nadir the FHR increases and temporarily "overshoots" and then returns to the baseline rate. Overshoots generally follow moderate and severe variable decelerations, have absent variability, and usually last more than 20 seconds.

Variable decelerations are frequently seen during the second stage of labor and are associated with stretching of the umbilical cord or compression of the cord as the fetus descends through the birth canal. Generally these can be tolerated by the fetus if the total time is short from the onset of decelerations to the time of delivery, as long as the baseline rate is not rising and variability is maintained (Freeman, Garite, Nageotte, 1991).

A progressively slower return to baseline with repetitive severe variable decelerations indicates a gradual increase in hypoxia. Severe uncorrectable variable decelerations, particularly with loss of variability and a rise in baseline rate are associated with fetal hypoxia, acidosis, and a neurologically depressed newborn.

The following summarizes and contrasts reassuring and nonreassuring variable decelerations (Freeman, Garite, Nageotte, 1991).

Reassuring Variable Decelerations	Nonreassuring Variable Decelerations
1. Last less than 30 to 45 seconds	1. <70 bpm for longer than >60 seconds
2. Abrupt rapid return to baseline	2. Prolonged return to baseline
3. Normal baseline rate continues	3. Increasing baseline rate
4. Variability does not decrease	4. Absence of variability

Intervention

Procedure*	Rationale
1. Change maternal position from side to side, Trendelenburg, or knee-chest	1. May relieve cord compression
2. When decelerations are severe:	2. Pattern may be a warning or nonreassuring sign
a. Discontinue oxytocin if infusing	a. Decreases UA, which can contribute to cord compression
b. Administer oxygen 8 to 10 L/min at 100% by snug face mask	b. Increases oxygen saturation of hemoglobin with maximum increase after about 9 minutes of 100% oxygen to the mother (McNamara, Johnson, Lilford, 1993)
c. Vaginal or speculum examination, or both	c. Assess for prolapsed umbilical cord or imminent delivery
d. Amnioinfusion, especially in the presence of oligohydramnios	d. Instillation of normal saline or lactated Ringer's solution through the intrauterine catheter may decrease frequency and severity of variable decelerations and relieve cord compression (see Chapter 7 for procedure)
e. Fetal oxygen saturation (FSpO$_2$) monitoring may	e. To distinguish normoxia from hypoxia in the fetus;

*Consider placement of internal electrode as appropriate for better assessment of potential problems.

Procedure	Rationale
be considered	values less than 30% indicates acidosis
f. Termination of labor is considered if the severe variable deceleration pattern cannot be corrected; if the pattern is corrected enough to be reassuring, the labor may be allowed to continue	f. Continuation of severe variable decelerations can only further compromise the fetus by increasing hypoxia and acidosis

Summary of Decelerations (Figure 6-7)

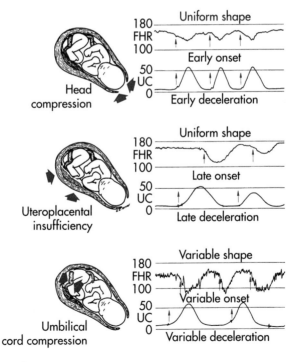

Figure 6-7
Summary of decelerations.

Early Declarations

ETIOLOGY	Head compression/vagal response
ONSET	Early; gradual; before peak of UC
RECOVERY	By end of contraction as uterine pressure returns to resting tone; gradual
DECELERATION	Rarely decelerates below 110 bpm
CLINICAL SIGNIFICANCE	Compensatory
NURSING INTERVENTION	Observe for changes of pattern, rate, and variability

Late Decelerations	Variable Decelerations
Uteroplacental insufficiency	Any interruption in umbilical blood flow; cord compression
Late; gradual; at or after peak of UC, with nadir, or low point, well after peak of UC	Variable; abrupt; anytime between or during contractions
After end of UC, well after pressure has returned to resting tone	Variable; may have rapid/abrupt return, prolonged return, shouldering over baseline (compensatory), or overshoot
Can decelerate any amount but is usually within normal FHR range of 110 to 160 bpm	Often decelerates below normal FHR range
Nonreassuring	May be transient; may progress to nonreassuring
Change maternal position	Change maternal position
Correct maternal hypotension; elevate legs; increase rate of maintenance IV infusion	Continue with the following only for nonreassuring variable decelerations:
Discontinue oxytocin if infusing	Discontinue oxytocin if infusing
Administer oxygen 8 to 10 L/min at 100% by snug face mask	Administer oxygen 8 to 10 L/min at 100% by snug face mask
Fetal scalp or acoustic stimulation, pH, fetal oxygen saturation ($FSpO_2$) monitoring; or termination of labor may be indicated	Vaginal or speculum examination, or both; amnioinfusion; fetal oxygen saturation ($FSpO_2$) monitoring; termination of labor may be indicated

Prolonged Deceleration
Definition

Prolonged deceleration of the fetal heart rate is a visually apparent decrease in FHR below the baseline. The decrease is determined from the most recently determined portion of the baseline. The decrease from the baseline is more than 15 bpm, lasting more than 2 minutes but less than 10 minutes from onset to return to baseline. A prolonged deceleration of more than 10 minutes is a baseline change (NICHD, 1997).

Description

Generally a prolonged deceleration is an isolated event. It is most frequently associated with occult or frank cord prolapse and progressive severe variable decelerations. It is characterized by a prolonged deceleration of 2 minutes or more and frequently decelerates below the average FHR range, although a tachycardic fetus may decelerate within the normal FHR range.

Characteristics (Figure 6-8)

SHAPE	Variable in shape; does not reflect the shape of any associated UC
ONSET	Variable times in the contracting phase
RECOVERY	May last 2 minutes or more, with a loss of variability and rebound tachycardia; occasionally a period of late decelerations follows; some fetuses do not recover, and the result is fetal death
DECELERATION	Deceleration is almost always below the normal FHR range except in a fetus with tachycardia
BASELINE	Often associated with a loss of variability and postdeceleration tachycardia
OCCURRENCE	Usually isolated events but may be seen late in the course of repetitive severe variable decelerations or during a prolonged series of late decelerations and just before fetal death

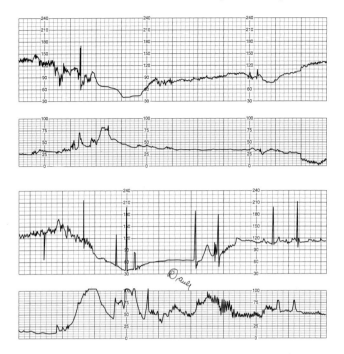

Figure 6-8
Prolonged decelerations.

Etiology

The causes and mechanisms of prolonged decelerations are listed.

Cause	Mechanism
1. Cord compression	1. A sudden occult or frank prolapse of umbilical cord
2. Maternal hypotension (supine or related to epidural or spinal anesthesia)	2. Profound uteroplacental insufficiency may result from hypotension, causing a prolonged deceleration

Cause	Mechanism
3. Paracervical anesthesia	3. Possibly related to fetal uptake of anesthetic agent, local hypotension from uterine artery spasms, or uterine hypertonus
4. Tetanic UCs (may be a result of oxytocin stimulation, abruptio placentae, epidural block, breast hyperstimulation, or cocaine ingestion)	4. Uterine tetany results in uteroplacental insufficiency; cocaine ingestion can result in vasospasm, hypertonus, and abruptio placenta; inadvertent IV injection of anesthetic with epidural block can result in a tetanic contraction and prolonged deceleration
5. Maternal hypoxia	5. Maternal seizure activity or respiratory depression (from narcotic overdose, magnesium sulfate toxicity, or high spinal anesthetic)
6. Procedures and physiological mechanisms: spiral electrode application; pelvic examination; sustained maternal Valsalva; rapid fetal descent through the birth canal	6. Fetal head compression/stimulation can produce a strong vagal response, cardiodeceleration, and prolonged deceleration

Clinical Significance

Prolonged deceleration(s) associated with fetal head compression (spiral electrode application, pelvic examination, sustained maternal Valsalva, rapid fetal descent) usually lasts for only 1 to 2 minutes and recovers with predeceleration variability and baseline. Decelerations caused by maternal hypotension, tetanic contractions, and maternal hypoxia generally occur with some loss of variability and tachycardia or recurrent late decelerations. If a subsequent prolonged deceleration does not recur, the placenta generally recovers the fetus to its predeceleration state. The prognosis for fetal survival is guarded if the prolonged deceleration occurs after a series of repetitive severe variable decelerations. In this situation, prolonged deceleration and/or recurrent late decelerations may result in a terminal bradycardia down to 30 to 60 bpm before death.

Intervention

Intervention is based on identifying and alleviating the cause of the prolonged variable deceleration. If the apparent cause is severe uteroplacental insufficiency or umbilical cord compression or is unidentifiable, then expeditious delivery may be indicated. Measures used to treat nonreassuring fetal status can be instituted in any case. These measures are described in detail in Chapter 7, "Assessment and Management of Fetal Status."

Lambda Pattern (Figure 6-9)

The lambda pattern is one that is common in early labor. It consists of an acceleration followed by a deceleration and then returns to baseline. The pattern is associated with uterine contractions. Typically appearing in early labor, this pattern does not persist (Freeman, Garite, Nageotte, 1991) and its physiology is unknown. This pattern does not require any intervention. It is included because it does occur at times and should not be confused with a late deceleration or other nonreassuring patterns.

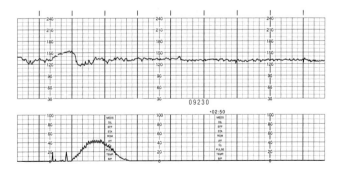

Figure 6-9
Lambda pattern.

Assessment and Management of Fetal Status

7

The focus of electronic fetal heart rate (FHR) monitoring during the intrapartum period is to identify the earliest stages of fetal hypoxia and then to intervene in an appropriate and timely manner to prevent fetal asphyxia, which can result from sustained and severe hypoxia. To do this, a knowledge of reassuring, concerning, and nonreassuring FHR patterns is essential to the implementation of appropriate interventions. Before reviewing these patterns it must be stated that there is no generally agreed upon precise definition of fetal distress. Hypoxia is considered to be a decreased level of oxygen in tissue below physiological levels, whereas asphyxia is the end result of profound hypoxia, resulting in anaerobic metabolism and resultant metabolic acidosis.

The diagnosis of birth asphyxia on the basis of fetal pH, Apgar score, and newborn cerebral dysfunction has been described by Gilstrap et al (1989) and the American College of Obstetricians and Gynecologists (ACOG, 1998a) and should only be applied in the clinical condition defined by the following:

1. Profound umbilical artery metabolic or mixed acidemia (pH <7.00, base deficit >20)
2. Persistence of an Apgar score of 0 to 3 for longer than 5 minutes
3. Neonatal neurological sequelae such as seizures, coma, and hypotonia
4. Multiorgan system dysfunction such as the cardiovascular, gastrointestinal, hematologic, renal, and/or pulmonary systems

When differentiating fetal stress from distress, variability is one of the major determinates that indicates the overall level of fetal oxygenation and fetal vigor. Variability is one way that the fetus exhibits its own ability to compensate and centralize oxygen. The presence of normal variability is associated with fetal vigor at birth (Parer, 1997). *Fetal stress* is evidenced by a change in the variability, baseline rate, or appearance of periodic and nonperiodic patterns that may be correctable by interventions such as maternal hydration, position change, and oxygenation.

Nonreassuring fetal status is a descriptive term that is used when the clinician who is interpreting the data is not reassured by the findings (ACOG, 1998a). The nonreassuring findings consist of a complete loss of variability, which may be accompanied by a change in baseline rate and may include the appearance of periodic and nonperiodic patterns (severe variable decelerations, late decelerations, or a bradycardia) that persist despite interventions. The presence of FHR variability indicates central nervous system and myocardial normoxia, whereas its decrease or absence in the presence of decelerations or bradycardia indicates a decrease in oxygenation to the central nervous system and myocardium (Parer, 1997). Diminished variability is secondary to a breakdown in the fetal compensatory mechanism to remain oxygenated. First, variability is lost within the periodic or nonperiodic changes. Next there is a progression to decreased, exaggerated (marked), or absent baseline variability or a sinusoidal pattern that without intervention or delivery may lead to fetal morbidity or mortality.

Research and experience suggest that a previously "normoxic" term fetus can tolerate late decelerations with variability present within the periodic change or severe variable decelerations for approximately 30 minutes before showing signs of decompensation. In light of this, it is crucial for all members of the obstetrical care delivery team to formulate and agree upon a plan of action for intervention before the end of a 30-minute period of nonreassuring FHR tracing *that has not been corrected or shown improvement as a result of interventions to enhance and optimize uteroplacental blood flow and fetal oxygenation* (Parer, 1997).

Several technologies exist and others are being developed and tested for the purpose of reducing intrapartum and antepartum risk to the pregnant woman and her fetus. For example, pulse oximetry used in labor as a means of measuring fetal oxygen saturation ($FSpO_2$) had been limited to experimental study and to limited clinical settings, until its recent approval for use in the United States to better assess a fetus with a nonreassuring FHR pattern.

As assessment tools are used and studied, a better understanding of the fetal response to stress (e.g., uterine contractions) has resulted. Literature and practitioners continue to disagree on the validity, efficacy, and cost effectiveness of surveillance tools and methods. This is due in part to the lack of agreement about definitions, labels, and parameters that warrant intervention. It is recommended that a chain of command and a plan be developed and agreed upon by the obstetrical medical, anesthetic, neonatal/ pediatric, nursing, and hospital administration staff for interventions for nonreassuring FHR patterns well before intervention is necessary (see Chapter 10 for "Chain of Command"). This plan should be based on accepted standards of care for the level of institution, resources, and personnel available in each care setting.

Although electronic fetal monitoring was intended to be used as a reflector of the adequacy of fetal oxygenation and not to reflect brain function, there are some FHR patterns that have been described as usually consistent with existing fetal brain damage. These include the following:

1. A flat tracing without late decelerations, variable decelerations, or prolonged bradycardia has been described with anencephaly (VanderMoer, Gerretsen, Visser, 1985 and Dicker et al, 1983).

2. A wandering pattern of blunt, slow, irregular undulations with a flat baseline has been reported with anencephaly (Freeman, Garite, Nageotte, 1991).

3. A sinusoidal electronic fetal monitoring pattern has been described in cases of hydrocephalus and severe anemia (Ombelet, VanDer Merwe, 1985; Parer, 1997).

4. A fixed heart rate with late decelerations and terminal bradycardias has been reported to occur in fetuses with severe central nervous system anomalies (Didolkar, Mutch, 1979).

Literature and practice suggest there is a consensus that an abnormal electronic fetal monitoring tracing is a poor predictor of cerebral palsy (CP), even though electronic fetal monitoring can help to identify fetal asphyxia, which can subsequently result in CP. Although this may seem contradictory, in reality (1) electronic fetal monitoring can fail to detect severe fetal asphyxia in an undetermined number of cases, (2) perinatal asphyxia is an uncommon cause of CP (possible causes include congenital developmental defects, intrauterine infection, intrauterine exposure to toxins and teratogens, hypothyroidism, and neonatal asphyxia [Hankins, 1991]), and (3) electronic fetal monitoring changes that reflect fetal asphyxia and/or acidosis may be the result of a damaged fetal brain and may be a consequence instead of the cause of CP (Niswander, 1991).

In conclusion, the focus of electronic FHR monitoring is to identify patterns that are reassuring and predictive of a positive fetal outcome. To do this, a knowledge of reassuring, concerning, and nonreassuring patterns is essential to prompt and appropriate interventions. This chapter describes patterns that are reassuring and considered normal, as well as concerning and nonreassuring patterns.

Assessment of Fetal Status

The fetal status should be assessed based on standards of practice and guidelines for patient care. The frequency of assessing fetal status during the intrapartum period follows (AAP/ACOG, 1997; AWHONN, 1997).

Stage of Labor	Low Risk	High Risk
Latent phase	q 30 to 60 minutes	q 30 minutes
Active phase	q 30 minutes	q 15 minutes
Second stage	q 15 minutes	q 5 minutes

The process of assessing fetal status during both the intrapartum and antepartum periods should be done in a thorough and systematic manner. The baseline FHR should be identified as being within the normal FHR range, tachycardia, or bradycardia. The amount of baseline variability should be assessed, noting the presence or absence of short-term variability and whether there is an undulating baseline. Periodic changes associated with uterine contractions and episodic or spontaneous changes should be noted, including accelerations and early, late, variable, or prolonged decelerations. Uterine activity should be assessed for the frequency and duration of contractions, and, if the patient is monitored by manual palpation, the strength and resting time should be noted. For patients being monitored internally with an intrauterine pressure catheter (IUPC), the intensity and resting tone in millimeters of mercury (mm Hg) pressure should be assessed. The following tool can be used as a checklist.

CHECKLIST FOR ASSESSMENT OF FETAL HEART RATE AND UTERINE ACTIVITY

1. What is the baseline fetal heart rate (FHR)?
   ___ Beats per minute (bpm)

   Check one of the following as observed on the tracing/monitor strip:
   ___ Average baseline FHR (normal range of 110 to 160 bpm)
   ___ Tachycardia (>160 bpm)
   ___ Bradycardia (<110 bpm)

2. What is the baseline variability?
   ___ Absent (range undetectable)
   ___ Minimal (>undetectable to ≤5 bpm)
   ___ Moderate (6 to 25 bpm)
   ___ Marked (>25 bpm)
   ___ Short-term variability: absent or present
   ___ Undulating baseline

3. Are there any periodic (associated with uterine contractions [UC]) or episodic (spontaneous) changes in the FHR?
   ___ Accelerations with fetal movement or stimulation
   ___ Accelerations with uterine contractions
   ___ Early decelerations (head compression)
   ___ Late decelerations (uteroplacental insufficiency)
   ___ Variable decelerations (cord compression)
       ___ Reassuring (<30 to 45 seconds, abrupt return to baseline, normal baseline rate, moderate variability)
       ___ Nonreassuring (>60 seconds, slow return to baseline, increasing baseline rate, absence of variability)
   ___ Prolonged deceleration (>15 bpm below baseline, >2 minutes to <10 minutes)

4. What is the uterine activity/contraction pattern (UA/UC)?
   ___ Frequency (onset to onset of UC)
   ___ Duration (beginning to end of contraction)

   Abdominal palpation method
   ___ Strength: mild, moderate, or strong
   ___ Resting time: from end of UC to start of next UC

   Internal monitoring/intrauterine pressure catheter
   ___ Intensity in mm Hg
   ___ Resting tone in mm Hg

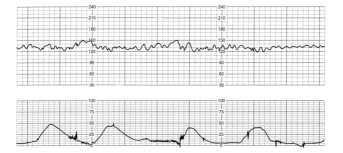

Figure 7-1
Average FHR and uterine activity pattern.

Reassuring Fetal Heart Rate Patterns

A reassuring fetal heart rate pattern (Figure 7-1) is one that is in the average FHR range of 110 to 160 bpm without tachycardia or bradycardia, demonstrates moderate (average) variability and the presence of short-term variability (STV) when electronically monitored, is reactive in that there are FHR accelerations with fetal movement, and exhibits an absence of late and nonreassuring variable decelerations (Berkus et al, 1999). Presence of variability throughout the baseline is indicative of a fetus with an intact autonomic nervous system and an ability to compensate for periods of stress.

Description

Baseline rate	110 to 160 bpm
Variability	Moderate ≥6 to ≤25 bpm; including presence of short-term variability
Periodic/episodic changes	None or accelerations with fetal movement, early decelerations, or reassuring variable decelerations

Normal Uterine Activity Pattern

FREQUENCY	More than 2 minutes between contractions
DURATION	Less than 90 seconds

INTENSITY   Less than 80 mm Hg pressure

RESTING TONE   Thirty seconds or more between contractions;
                 resting intrauterine pressure less than 20 mm
                 Hg (can be determined only by intrauterine
                 monitoring)

A reassuring FHR and uterine activity pattern serves to allay the concerns of the patient and staff about the fetal status during labor. This reassuring type of pattern indicates that the fetus is tolerating the process of labor well and does not require any type of intervention. One would expect to have a good fetal outcome with normal Apgar scores and blood gases.

Concerning Fetal Heart Rate Patterns

Concerning FHR patterns may be self-limiting or they may proceed and lead to nonreassuring FHR patterns. If the recording of these patterns is not clear or is of poor quality or if a more accurate assessment of the pattern is necessary, consider the direct method of monitoring with a spiral electrode until the pattern becomes reassuring or until intervention for a nonreassuring pattern is indicated. Concerning patterns include the following:

- Progressive increase/decrease or shift in baseline FHR
- Tachycardia of 160 bpm or more
- Decreasing baseline variability without any identified cause (e.g., narcotics)

Nonreassuring Fetal Heart Rate Patterns and Interventions (Figures 7-2, 7-3, and 7-4)

Nonreassuring FHR patterns are those characterized by loss of variability and periodic and nonperiodic or episodic FHR changes. These include severe variable decelerations, late decelerations, absence of variability, prolonged decelerations, severe bradycardia, and sinusoidal patterns. These patterns are associated with metabolic or respiratory acidosis or both and when uncorrected may lead to fetal morbidity or mortality (Table 7-1).

The primary goal of interventions for nonreassuring patterns is to enhance fetal oxygenation as reflected by a conversion to a reassuring FHR pattern. The physiological goals of the interventions are intended to improve uterine blood flow, umbilical circulation,

Text continued on p. 136

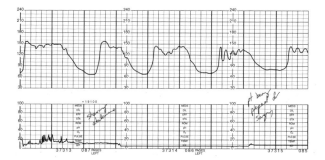

Figure 7-2
Nonreassuring FHR pattern: Severe variable decelerations with flat baseline.

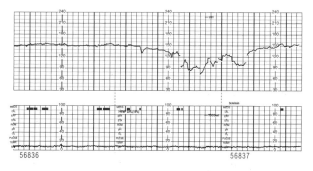

Figure 7-3
Nonreassuring FHR pattern: Spontaneous (nonperiodic) prolonged deceleration.

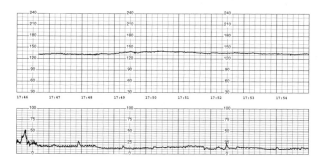

Figure 7-4
Nonreassuring pattern: Absence of variability.

Table 7-1   Identification and Management of Nonreassuring
FHR Patterns

Nonreassuring Fetal Heart Rate Patterns	Intervention
Severe variable deceleration FHR nadir below 70 bpm, lasting longer than 60 seconds with any of the following:	With severe variable deceleration: Change maternal position
Rising baseline FHR Decreasing variability Slow return to baseline	Perform vaginal or speculum examination, or both
	Discontinue oxytocin if infusing (consider tocolysis)
	Administer oxygen at 8 to 10 L/min at 100% by snug face mask
	Amnioinfusion may be considered (see p. 149)
	Increase rate of maintenance IV infusion
	Fetal oxygen saturation (FSpO$_2$) monitoring may be considered (see p. 140)
	Termination of labor should be considered if pattern cannot be corrected enough to meet criteria of mild deceleration
Late decelerations of any magnitude, more serious if associated with decreasing variability or rising baseline	Intervene in step-by-step approach, proceeding to next step if pattern is uncorrected

Purpose	Rationale
To relieve pressure on the umbilical cord	Improves and optimizes umbilical and uteroplacental blood flow
To rule out a prolapsed cord	Continue other interventions or set p for emergent cesarean delivery if cord is prolapsed
To reduce repetitive pressure on cord and decrease uterine hyperstimulation	Discontinue exogenous source of uterine stimulation
To promote maternal hyperoxia	Increases fetal oxygen saturation ($FSpO_2$)
To relieve pressure on the umbilical cord by adding fluid to "cushion" cord	Correct oligohydramnios
To correct maternal hypotension and reverse dehydration	Increases circulating blood volume
To distinguish normoxia from hypoxia in the fetus	A value less than 30% indicates acidosis
To decrease stress/hypoxia on fetus	Fetal position, stage of labor, dilatation, and effacement should be considered in continuance of labor in the presence of a nonreassuring FHR pattern

Continued

Table 7-1   Identification and Management of Nonreassuring
FHR Patterns—cont'd

Nonreassuring Fetal Heart Rate Patterns	Intervention
Late decelerations—continued	Place patient in lateral position
	Lower head of bed
	Increase rate of maintenance IV infusion
	Discontinue oxytocin if infusing (do this first if uterine hyperstimulation is present); consider tocolysis
	Administer oxygen at 8 to 10 L/min at 100% by snug face mask
	Stimulate fetal scalp or give sound stimulation
	Fetal oxygen saturation ($FSpO_2$) monitoring may be considered (see p. 140)
Absence of variability	Correct identifiable cause; consider $FSpO_2$ monitoring; administer maternal oxygen
Prolonged deceleration	As above
Severe bradycardia	As above
Sinusoidal pattern	As above

See discussion of tocolysis therapy for nonreassuring fetal heart rate patterns
(p. 153).

Purpose	Rationale
To correct supine hypotension and improve uterine blood flow	Removes the weight of the fetus from the inferior vena cava, which then allows better blood return to the heart, increasing maternal cardiac output and subsequently blood pressure
To correct maternal hypotension	Diminishes pooling of blood in extremities and increases circulating volume
To correct maternal hypotension and reverse dehydration	Increases circulating blood volume
To reduce uterine activity	Decreases strength and frequency of uterine contractions, which can improve uteroplacental blood flow
To promote maternal hyperoxia	Increases fetal oxygen saturation ($FSpO_2$)
To identify FHR reactivity and produce acceleration; gives indication of fetal oxygenation and pH	Indicates fetal well-being; if the fetus is able to produce accelerations, it shows ability to compensate; pH is generally >7.2
To distinguish normoxia from hypoxia in the fetus	Values less than 30% indicates acidosis
To determine if result of narcotic administration, position, uterine hyperstimulation, rapid descent, cord prolapse, abruption, uterine rupture, fetal anomaly, or prolonged uteroplacental insufficiency	To determine if cause is reversible or changeable; document event, notify appropriate OB team members, and, if warranted, prepare for immediate delivery

Mixed (or Combination) Fetal Heart Rate Patterns

The following are examples of mixed FHR patterns:
1. Early and variable decelerations
2. Early and late decelerations
3. Late and variable decelerations
4. Prolonged deceleration following any other deceleration

In mixed patterns the potential fetal compromise associated with the FHR pattern should be evaluated by the most nonreassuring component of the pattern, such as absent baseline variability or late decelerations. This then provides the direction for appropriate interventions.

and oxygenation and to reduce uterine activity (AWHONN, 1997). The interventions are sometimes referred to as *intrauterine resuscitation* and include maternal position change, hydration, maternal oxygen, amnioinfusion for cord compression, a decrease or discontinuance of uterine stimulant medications, tocolysis, or other medications. When efforts fail to convert the fetal status to a reassuring one, the interventions should continue to optimize fetal oxygenation until such time that delivery is effected. The preceding Table 7-1 lists the specific interventions based on the type of nonreassuring pattern, their purposes, and their rationales.

Other Methods of Assessment/Intervention

The primary hypothesis for intrapartum surveillance is the timely identification of and intervention for the hypoxic or acidotic fetus to prevent intrauterine death and decrease long-term neurological damage and sequelae (Yoon et al, 1993). Studies show that most accurate assessments of fetal well-being and degree of asphyxia are best determined when electronic fetal monitoring is used in conjunction with other tools. Some tools of assessment are used during the intrapartum period and others after delivery to reconstruct hypoxic episodes. To date, $FSpO_2$ monitoring appears to be the most optimal method to identify fetal hypoxia during the intrapartum period.

Fetal Heart Rate Response to Stimulation

Stimulation of the fetus to elicit an acceleration of FHR for at least 15 seconds has been reported as an alternative to scalp pH testing, a discussion of which is found in the next section. Several studies have correlated the fetal scalp pH with the FHR response to a stimulus and have attested to the efficacy of these mechanisms. Stimulation methods include the following:

1. *Scalp stimulation:* Digital pressure and rubbing of the scalp for 15 seconds, followed by application of an atraumatic Allis clamp to the scalp for 15 seconds
2. *Sound stimulation:* Vibroacoustic stimulation (VAS) by placing an artificial larynx on the maternal abdomen over the fetal head

The rationale for use of these mechanisms is that if an acceleration of 15 bpm for 15 seconds occurs with the stimulation in a fetus beyond 32 weeks' gestation (or 10 bpm for 10 seconds if fetus ≤32 weeks), one can assume that the fetal pH is normal. Studies have shown that no less than 50% of stimulated fetuses will have an FHR acceleration, and this is highly predictive of fetal well-being and a pH of no less than 7.25. Of the fetuses that do not accelerate, about one half are not acidotic; therefore absence of an acceleration to the stimulus is not totally predictive of an abnormal pH, fetal acidosis, or fetal distress.

Fetal Blood Sampling for Acid-Base Monitoring

Fetal blood sampling (Figure 7-5) was first described by Saling in 1962 as a means of identifying fetal hypoxemia and acidosis. When the fetus is faced with hypoxia, metabolism changes from aerobic to anaerobic. This results in the production of lactic acid and a subsequent drop in pH. Therefore a decrease in blood pH becomes a measure of the degree of hypoxia.

Thus fetal scalp sampling was developed as a means of identifying the degree of fetal hypoxia at the time of testing. Studies show that many variables can lead to false elevations or drops in results. This form of assessment is not usually a standard of practice in all institutions unless opportunities exist for development of technique and proper equipment for testing is readily available on site. In fact, because of its invasive nature, high rate of inaccurate results, and delay in obtaining results, this technique is no longer used in the majority of the perinatal units in the United States (Simpson, 1998).

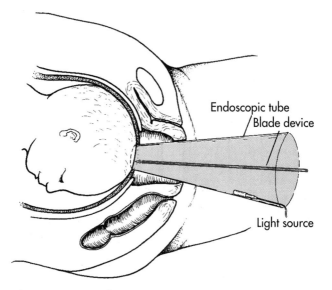

Figure 7-5
Schema of fetal blood sampling.

Samples are usually collected aerobically and in small amounts. If the samples are difficult to obtain or the drops of blood are slow forming, the results may show falsely elevated pH values. Fetal scalp sampling is invasive, and initiation of sampling usually requires repeated sampling every 15 to 30 minutes to monitor pH values.

A small amount of fetal blood is obtained from the skin of the presenting part—usually the fetal scalp. To measure Po_2, Pco_2, and base deficit, a larger sample of fetal blood is required. Because these values do not provide enough additional information to warrant their measurement, and because blood gas values can vary so rapidly with transient circulatory changes, the use of fetal blood sampling during the intrapartum period is not routinely warranted. Measurements vary during different stages of labor. Various factors can influence pH during the intrapartum/predelivery period and make values disproportionate to the condition at birth. These factors are listed as follows:

1. Maternal acidosis or alkalosis
2. Laboratory errors or delay in determination

3. Caput succedaneum (↓ pH value)
4. Stage of labor
5. Time relationship of scalp sampling to uterine contractions
6. Influence of in utero treatment
7. Transience of the insult causing fetal acidosis (metabolic acidosis is less readily reversible than respiratory acidosis)
8. Contamination of sample with amniotic fluid (↓ pH value) or room air (↑ pH value)
9. Contamination with meconium

Interpretation of Values

The normal range of pH in an adult is 7.35 to 7.45. The average fetal range is 7.30 to 7.35, with values above 7.25 considered normal. A value between 7.20 and 7.25 is considered preacidotic, and the blood sample is usually repeated within 15 to 30 minutes to detect the possibility of a downward trend. A scalp blood pH of less than 7.20 is considered frank acidosis and indicates the need for some type of medical or surgical intervention (Freeman, Garite, Nageotte, 1991).

Normal fetal scalp values

pH	7.25 to 7.35
Po_2	20-30 mm Hg
Pco_2	40 to 50 mm Hg
Base deficit	<10 mEq/L

Anaerobic metabolism will occur in the fetus in the absence of oxygen, resulting in the production of lactic acid, which accumulates to lower the fetal pH and thus serves as an indirect measure of fetal oxygenation. When respiratory acidosis occurs in the fetus, as can occur with cord compression demonstrated by variable decelerations, the pH is low, the Pco_2 markedly elevated, and the base deficit usually unchanged. With metabolic acidosis caused by uteroplacental insufficiency and demonstrated by late decelerations, the pH is low, the Po_2 decreased, the Pco_2 mildly elevated, and the base deficit elevated (possibly exceeding 10 to 15 mEq/L).

The role of lactate measurements from the fetal scalp during labor using a microvolume lactate meter has been studied. Comparison between lactate and pH in scalp blood revealed a significant correlation. The blood sampling procedures were more successful and required fewer scalp incisions per blood sampling attempts. Additional clinical management trials may determine the clinical usefulness of this method and how it should be combined with other modalities for fetal monitoring (Westgren, Kublickas, Kruger, 1999; Kruger, Kublickas, Westgren, 1998).

Umbilical Cord Acid-Base Determination

A useful adjunct to the Apgar score in assessing the immediate condition of the newborn is to obtain a sample of cord blood. It may be helpful to rule out asphyxia in the presence of a low Apgar score. If metabolic acidosis is not present, then it is not likely that the low Apgar score is caused by intrapartum asphyxia.

The procedure consists of double-clamping a 10- to 20-cm (approximately 4 to 8 inches) segment of the umbilical cord immediately after delivery of the infant. A specimen should be drawn with a 1-ml plastic syringe that has been flushed with heparin solution (1000 U/ml). Draw blood from the umbilical artery or, if that is not possible, from the umbilical vein. Separate syringes should be used if drawing blood from both the umbilical vein and umbilical artery. Normal values for cord blood are summarized as follows (ACOG, 1995c; Helwig, 1996):

Normal values for umbilical cord blood

Cord Blood	pH	P_{CO_2} (mm Hg)	P_{O_2} (mm Hg)	Bicarbonate (mEq/L)
Arterial	7.27	53.0	17.0	22.3
(range)	(7.15-7.43)	(31.1-74.3)	(3.8-33.8)	(13.3-27.5)
Venous	7.35	41.0	29.0	20.4
(range)	(7.24-7.49)	(23.2-49.2)	(15.4-48.2)	(15.9-24.7)

Fetal Oxygen Saturation Monitoring

Fetal oxygen saturation ($FSpO_2$) monitoring is the most significant change in intrapartum fetal assessment since the introduction of FHR monitoring and fetal scalp sampling 30 years ago (Dildy, Clark, Loucks, 1996). The primary value of fetal oxygenation saturation ($FSpO_2$) monitoring is to better assess fetal status in the presence of a nonreassuring FHR pattern as observed during electronic FHR monitoring. The value obtained reliably identifies the fetus who is adequately oxygenated from the fetus who is not. This information then provides the direction for clinical management as to either the continuation of labor or the need for intervention.

Intended Use for Fetal Oxygen Saturation Monitoring

Fetal oxygen saturation ($FSpO_2$) monitoring is a tool to be used in conjunction with an electronic FHR monitor to provide data that result in a more complete picture of fetal status. It is designed to be used when the fetus presents a nonreassuring FHR tracing. After insertion the sensor can remain in place throughout the remainder of the labor and unassisted vaginal delivery. The sensor must be removed for vacuum extraction, forceps delivery, or cesarean delivery.

Contraindications

Fetal oxygen saturation ($FSpO_2$) monitoring cannot be used for patients who are not in labor nor when membranes are intact. Patients with the following conditions are not candidates: documented placenta previa, low-lying placenta, placental abruption, vaginal bleeding of unknown origin, uterine anomalies, presence of intrauterine or vaginal infection, such as beta-streptococcal infection, active genital herpes simplex infection, or any other infection that precludes internal monitoring.

Description and Mechanism of Pulse Oximetry Technology

The fetal oxygen saturation ($FSpO_2$) monitor measures functional oxygen saturation of arterial hemoglobin ($FSpO_2$) and detects the fetal pulse rate via a flexible-tipped reflectance sensor that is placed against the fetal cheek in a gentle nontraumatic way. Traditionally, the typical method of monitoring used on adult/pediatric/neonatal (ex utero) patients has been a transmission type of sensor in which the optical components are positioned opposite each other so that light passes through the tissue of a finger, toe, or ear or across the bridge of the nose from one side to the other (Figure 7-6, *A*). The fetal oximeter differs in that it uses a reflectance sensor in which the optical components are on the same monitoring surface. The light-emitting diodes (LEDs) on the sensor shine light into tissue, and the photodetector measures the light back-scattering, that is, the reflection of light coming out of the tissue (Figure 7-6, *B*).

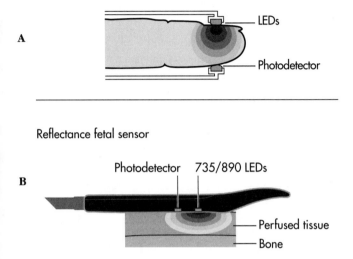

Figure 7-6
Pulse oximetry sensors. **A,** Maternal sensor; optical components are positioned opposite each other and light passes through. **B,** Fetal sensor; optical components are positioned on the same side and light is reflected back from the tissue.
(Courtesy Mallinckrodt, Inc., Pleasanton, Calif.)

The same basic principles of physics apply to both conventional (ex utero) and fetal pulse oximetry; however, a different wavelength for the red LED is used to assess the low levels of oxygen saturation that are seen in the fetus, contrasted with the adult. Typically, fetal oxygen saturation ($FSpO_2$) is normally between 30% and 70% during labor, whereas the saturation of the extrauterine patient is generally 95% to 100%. Through years of clinical study it was determined that the use of a different wavelength for the red LED would optimize the system for fetal use.

Pulse oximetry works on the principle that well-oxygenated blood looks bright red compared with poorly oxygenated blood. On the front surface of the fetal sensor are two LEDs of different

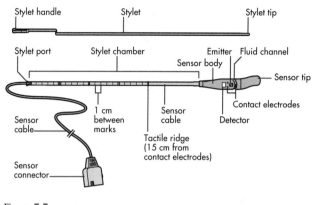

Figure 7-7
Nellcor fetal oxygen sensor (illustration) with key points
identified.
(Courtesy Mallinckrodt, Inc., Pleasanton, Calif.)

wavelengths (Figure 7-7). One LED is red and the other is infrared. The red light is absorbed more by deoxyhemoglobin (dark
blood), and the infrared light is absorbed more by oxyhemoglobin
(bright red blood). The photodetector captures the light that is reflected back from the tissue (the blood in the tissues of the fetal
cheek). The difference in the amount of light that is emitted by the
LEDs versus the amount that is reflected back represents the
amount of light that is absorbed by both the oxyhemoglobin and
deoxyhemoglobin. It is this difference that is used in the determination of fetal oxygen saturation. The greater the ratio of red to infrared, the lower the oxygen saturation and vice versa (Dildy,
Clark, Loucks, 1996).

Monitoring Equipment

The Nellcor N-400 fetal oxygen saturation ($FSpO_2$) monitoring
system (Mallinckrodt, Inc., Pleasanton, Calif.) is currently the only
system that has undergone multicenter, randomized, controlled
clinical trials. The Nellcor FS-14 Series Fetal Oxygen Sensor (Figure 7-8) can only be used with the Nellcor N-400 Fetal Oxygen
Saturation Monitor (Figure 7-9) or with an electronic fetal monitor
containing patented Nellcor technology. Fetal monitors containing
the integrated Nellcor technology include the Agilent Technologies

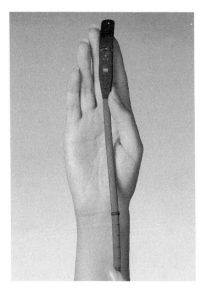

Figure 7-8
Nellcor FS-14 Series fetal oxygen sensor.
(Courtesy Mallinkrodt, Inc., Pleasanton, Calif.)

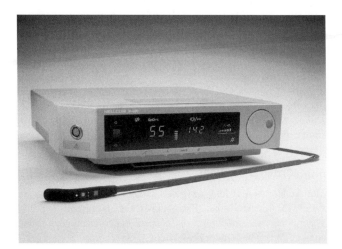

Figure 7-9
The Nellcor N-400 Fetal Oxygen Saturation Monitor can
interface with a fetal monitor with a connecting cable. The
FSpO$_2$ will trace on the uterine activity panel of the tracing.
(Courtesy Mallinkrodt, Inc., Pleasanton, Calif.)

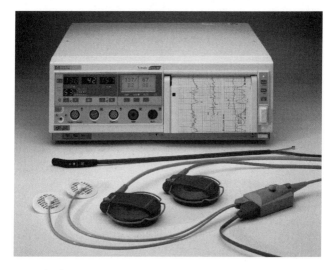

Figure 7-10
Viridia 50XMO Fetal Maternal Monitor with port for Nellcor
Sensor FS-14 to monitor FSpO₂.
(Courtesy Agilent Technologies, Böblingen, Germany).

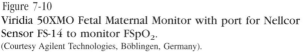

Viridia Series XMO (Figure 7-10) and the Corometrics 120 Series
fetal monitors (models 126, 128, and 129). The fetal sensor cord
plugs into the outlet on the face of these fetal monitors, and the fetal oxygen saturation is displayed on the monitor screen. Interface
capabilities using a special cable that connects the fetal monitor
with the N-400 fetal oximeter are available on some older fetal
monitors, including the Corometrics model 118, Hewlett Packard
(HP) model 8040A, Viridia Series 50 IP, and the Meridian Sonic-
aid 800 monitor.

Whether the fetal oxygen saturation ($FSpO_2$) monitor is inter-
faced with a fetal monitor or integrated into the fetal monitor, the
technology provides for simultaneous documentation of fetal oxygen saturation, uterine activity, and FHR on the same tracing. Fetal
oxygen saturation values are recorded as a nearly continuous line
on the uterine activity area of the chart paper (Figure 7-11). These
two parameters are conveniently recorded together because both
are measured on a 1- to 100-unit scale.

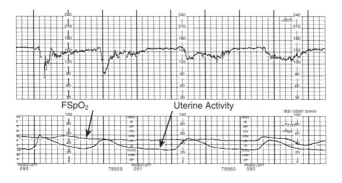

Figure 7-11
Note FSpO$_2$ tracing on uterine activity panel of fetal
monitoring strip.
(Courtesy Mallinkrodt, Inc., Pleasanton, Calif.)

Requirements for Sensor Insertion

For sensor insertion the amniotic membranes must be ruptured and
the cervix must be adequately dilated to at least 2 cm. Rupturing
the membranes with the sensor should not be attempted. The fetal
head must be sufficiently descended into the pelvis that the sensor
is held by natural pressures against the fetal face, which is at least
a minus two station. Candidates for this technology are essentially
those patients in labor who demonstrate nonreassuring FHR patterns and who are candidates for the internal mode of electronic
FHR monitoring.

Fetal Sensor Placement and Position

As an intrauterine device the fetal oximetry sensor is inserted in a
similar manner as the intrauterine pressure catheter, with some no-
table differences. The sensor is not advanced into the uterine cavity nearly as far as the IUPC, and the process for insertion and
placement on the optimum location is a learned skill based on the
manufacturer's directions. The procedure for insertion of the sensor is initiated with an examination of the presenting part. After
identifying the sagittal suture and one or both of the fontanels, the
sensor is introduced between uterine contractions. The fetal oximetry sensor is a flexible probe that is inserted through the cervical
os and comes to lie alongside the cheek and temple area of the fe-

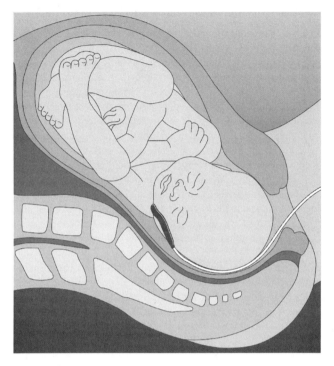

Figure 7-12
Placement and position of FSpO$_2$ sensor.
(Courtesy Mallinkrodt, Inc., Pleasanton, Calif.)

tal face (Figure 7-12). This is the optimal site for monitoring because fetal pulses tend to be larger in this area and artifact problems that can be caused by hair, vernix, caput, and venous stasis are not typically encountered. The fulcrum tip design of the sensor helps to hold it in place by the natural pressures that are present in the labor process. As labor progresses the sensor generally descends and rotates with the presenting part. On occasion, a minor adjustment to sensor position may be required. A complete and detailed description of the sensor placement technique can be found in the Nellcor FS-14 Series Fetal Oxygen Sensor Placement Guide.

Critical Threshold Value for Fetal Oxygen Saturation

The basic interpretation model for fetal oxygen saturation ($FSpO_2$) depends on the existence of a critical threshold value for fetal oxygen saturation that reliably separates the fetus who is adequately oxygenated from the fetus who is not. Both animal and human studies support the existence of a critical threshold value for fetal oxygen saturation at 30% based on the correlation of fetal oxygen saturation with fetal scalp pH during labor. The critical threshold accurately predicts intrapartum acidosis defined as a fetal scalp pH <7.20 with an 81% sensitivity and 100% specificity (Kühnert, Seelback-Goebel, Butterwegge, 1998). Additionally, it was found that oxidative metabolism cannot be maintained when the fetal oxygen saturation remains lower than 30% for 10 minutes or more because this results in a progressive fall in pH and extracellular fluid base excess (Swedlow, 1998). Low fetal arterial oxygen saturation data <30% for at least 10 minutes or longer correlate significantly with low scalp pH values and have a predictive value with regard to fetal outcome (Kühnert, Seelback-Goebel, Butterwegge, 1998). Fetal oxygen saturation is more predictive of fetal status than scalp sampling for fetal pH because of the various factors such as caput formation and venous stasis that can influence pH values during the intrapartum/predelivery period.

Interpretation and Management

A written clinical management protocol utilizing research-based recommendations and guidelines should be in place in each institution using fetal pulse oximetry technology. General guidelines for interpretation and management that follow are based on information from randomized clinical trials in the United States (Dildy et al, 1997) and studies and use of fetal oxygen saturation in Europe (Kühnert et al, 1998).

A fetal oxygen saturation ($FSpO_2$) value in excess of 30% is considered reassuring, and labor is generally allowed to continue unless otherwise indicated by the physician. A value less than 30% is considered nonreassuring, and conventional interventions for nonreassuring FHR patterns should be implemented while continuing to observe the pattern over a 10-minute period. The interventions include maternal position change, correction of maternal hypotension, improvement of maternal hydration, amnioinfusion, reduction or discontinuance of oxytocic drugs, administration of tocolytics, and administration of supplemental oxygen at 8 to 10

L/min by snug face mask. Confirmation of fetal acidosis with scalp pH can be obtained if scalp sampling is readily available. If the fetal oxygen saturation remains less than 30% for longer than 10 minutes, the physician may perform an expeditious delivery using forceps, vacuum extraction, or cesarean delivery. The choice of delivery technique should be based on the condition of the mother and fetus, the stage of labor, the pressure of time, and the skill of the provider (Kühnert et al, 1998).

Fetal pulse oximetry is a promising new method of fetal assessment. It is anticipated that cesarean deliveries done for nonreassuring FHR patterns can be reduced significantly with the knowledge of a reassuring fetal oxygen saturation ($FSpO_2$) value (Dildy et al, 1997, 2000). The contribution of better methods of fetal assessment to decrease unnecessary interventions will be a major improvement in the provision of quality perinatal care (Simpson, 1998).

Intervention for Fetal Distress
Amnioinfusion

Amnioinfusion is a procedure used to replace amniotic fluid with normal saline or lactated Ringer's solution through the intrauterine pressure catheter. With the advent of amnioinfusion, fetal stress may be decreased and the chances for a vaginal delivery are increased (Wallerstedt et al, 1994). Amnioinfusion is an effective technique used to reduce variable decelerations caused by cord compression and to reduce the incidence of meconium aspiration in the presence of thick meconium (Miyasaki, Taylor, 1983; Miyasaki, Nevarez, 1985).

Patients with documented oligohydramnios (secondary to uteroplacental insufficiency, premature rupture of membranes, or postmaturity) are at risk for developing cord compression. Cord compression is evidenced by variable decelerations during labor. With oligohydramnios, when the uterus contracts the cord becomes more vulnerable to compression. Amnioinfusion replaces the "cushion" for the cord and relieves both the frequency and intensity of variable decelerations.

Another indication for amnioinfusion is the presence of moderate to thick ("pea soup") meconium. The presence or absence of meconium is now known to be a reliable indicator of the amount of fetal stress during labor (Berkus et al, 1994). It is estimated that 12% of all fetuses pass meconium before delivery. At approximately 36 weeks' gestation, the fetus excretes motilin into the intestine, which facilitates peristalsis. Therefore the presence of meconium before 36 weeks' gestation is unusual. In the presence of fetal hypoxia the anal sphincter relaxes and intestinal peristalsis increases, facilitating the passage of meconium in utero. Many fetuses who have meconium in their amniotic fluid at delivery do not show signs of hypoxia. However, the passage of meconium late in labor in association with FHR abnormalities has been shown to be a warning sign of possible fetal distress. The asphyxiated fetus gasps in utero and inhales meconium into the large airways. If meconium is not removed from these airways at birth (before the neonate's first breaths), the meconium is pulled into the distal airways and air is trapped in the alveoli, resulting in inadequate airway exchange (meconium aspiration syndrome).

Intrapartum patients with meconium present are considered to be high risk, and the FHR pattern should be continually assessed, with timely and appropriate interventions performed if nonreassuring patterns are identified. The purpose of amnioinfusion in the presence of moderate to thick meconium is to dilute and flush out the meconium. Studies show that when amnioinfusion has been used for the presence of meconium, Apgar scores are higher, the incidence of operative delivery is decreased, and less meconium is visualized below the vocal cords during intubation and suctioning (Wallerstedt et al, 1994).

To ensure that meconium is not aspirated by the neonate, special care should be taken during the delivery process. The nasopharynx and oropharynx should be suctioned immediately as the head is being delivered. The mother may need to be instructed to blow repetitively to refrain from pushing to allow for suctioning to occur before the neonate takes its first breath. Following delivery the neonate, if not vigorous, should be subject to endotracheal intubation and tracheal suctioning until the meconium is cleared. All of these procedures should be clearly described in the patient's record by the person performing them.

Saline has been found to be the replacement fluid most resembling amniotic fluid; however, lactated Ringer's solution can also be used. One risk to this intervention is the potential for iatrogenic polyhydramnios. It is critical to accurately assess fluid output during amnioinfusion and to monitor for increases in uterine resting tone. Infusion pumps or gravity flow can be used to deliver the amnioinfusion solution. Documentation of total amount administered and any other complications that occur is imperative. Placental detachment may be the result of overdistention of the uterus secondary to iatrogenic polyhydramnios.

Theoretically, in the presence of abruptio placentae, the risk of fluid emboli is increased with the use of amnioinfusion. Umbilical cord prolapse with amnioinfusion is another possible concern if the presenting part is not engaged in the pelvic inlet. The saline solution used for amnioinfusion is generally at room temperature for term infants or warmed to body temperature only by blood warmer if the fetus is preterm. Amnioinfusion solution should **never** be warmed in the microwave or in a blanket warmer.

Indications

1. Laboring preterm patients with premature rupture of the membranes
2. Patients with otherwise uncorrectable variable decelerations during labor
3. Known cases of significant oligohydramnios (amniotic fluid index ≤5) at term when undergoing induction of labor
4. Presence of moderate to thick ("pea soup") meconium

Equipment and supplies

1. 1000 ml normal saline or lactated Ringer's solution (at room temperature)
2. Internal uterine catheter equipment, preferably with a double lumen or amnioport
3. IV extension tubing with twin sites or arterial line (12 inches) and a four-way stopcock if needed
4. Volumetric infusion pump and tubing or IV pole for gravity flow
5. Blood warmer or blood fluid warming set (optional)

NOTE: When the fetus is preterm and the procedure is being done prophylactically, a warming unit or preferred solution warmed to body temperature (98.6° F) should be used.

Preprocedure

1. Place patient in a lateral position
2. Administer 100% oxygen by snug face mask 8 to 10 L/min as indicated by assessment of monitor tracing
3. Continuously monitor the patient

Procedure

This procedure should be initiated after insertion of the intrauterine catheter. Before the procedure the intrauterine resting tone should be noted with the patient in the right and left lateral and the supine position for later comparison.

1. Connect 1000 ml of amnioinfusion solution to IV tubing.
2. Flush tubing with solution.
3. Connect tubing to patient's intrauterine pressure catheter (IUPC) via amnioport, or double-lumen IUPC, or via a three-way stopcock as indicated based on type of IUPC used.
4. Initiate the flow of amnioinfusion and instill the initial bolus, usually 250 to 600 ml over a 15- to 60-minute period (10 to 15 ml/min) using either an infusion pump or gravity flow. If gravity flow is used, the solution must be hung about 3 to 4 feet above the level of the tip of the IUPC.
5. When variable decelerations resolve, continue the infusion at a slower rate, usually about 2 to 3 ml/min (120 to 180 ml/hr), as ordered by the care provider. If variable decelerations are not relieved after infusing 800 to 1000 ml of solution, the procedure may be discontinued and alternative interventions performed.

NOTE: Intrauterine resting tone will appear higher than normal, from 25 to 40 mm Hg because of resistance to outflow through the tiny holes in the tip of the catheter. The true resting tone can be checked by temporarily discontinuing the flow of infusion.

Patient care

Care of the patient undergoing amnioinfusion includes the following:

1. Stop the infusion periodically, approximately every 30 minutes, to note the baseline uterine pressure. Notify the physician if the resting tone is greater than 25 mm Hg to evaluate continuation of the procedure.
2. Change the underpads frequently to ensure patient comfort. This is necessary because of the increase in vaginal fluid leakage.
3. Note the color and amount of fluid on the underpad. The underpad may be weighed. Amounts of fluid returned should be determined. One milliliter of fluid equals approximately 1 gram of weight.
4. Monitor patient for signs and symptoms of infection.
5. Monitor for signs and symptoms of cardiac or respiratory com-

promise. An overexpanded uterus pressing on the diaphragm may cause maternal shortness of breath, hypotension, or tachycardia.

6. Monitor for concerning or nonreassuring fetal patterns on the electronic fetal monitoring strip. Fetal bradycardia may occur if the solution is cold and is infused rapidly.

Intrapartal Tocolysis Therapy for Nonreassuring Fetal Heart Rate Patterns

Although tocolytic therapy is routinely used to prevent and manage preterm labor, it can be used as an adjunct to other interventions in the management of nonreassuring FHR patterns. When the fetus is exhibiting signs of stress with concomitant increased uterine activity that is not responsive to position change and discontinuance of the oxytocin infusion, an intravenous or subcutaneous injection of terbutaline can be administered while preparation for immediate delivery is in process. A cesarean delivery may be performed if the nonreassuring FHR pattern persists and the fetus cannot be safely delivered vaginally. Conversely, if the FHR pattern improves, then the patient may be allowed to continue labor. Terbutaline, which has a shorter time of onset, is generally preferred to magnesium sulfate, which has a longer time of onset. If the patient delivers shortly after the administration of terbutaline, there is a risk of uterine atony and postpartum hemorrhage. Therefore appropriate preparations should be made if delivery appears imminent.

Nitroglycerin, a potent smooth muscle relaxant and vasodilator, has been used for acute tocolysis on selected patients for indications such as shoulder dystocia, acute hypertonus with fetal distress, head entrapment of preterm infants, delivery of the head in difficult cesarean and breech deliveries, and persistent bradycardia during set-up for cesarean delivery. It has been administered by aerosol sublingual spray, sublingual tablet, transdermal patch, and intravenously. Nitroglycerin (glyceryl trinitrate) can cause hypotension and compensatory sympathetic responses leading to tachycardia; therefore it is used very selectively in order to effect uterine relaxation for acute tocolysis (Black, 1999).

Intrapartal Tocolytic Drugs

Any one of the following may be ordered by the physician to effect a reduction in uterine activity (Brown, 1998; ACOG, 1995e;

Valenzuela, Foster, 1990; Burke et al, 1989; Garite, Ray, 1988; Arias, 1978):

1. Terbutaline 0.125 to 0.25 mg by slow IV push (1 minute)
2. Terbutaline 0.25 mg subcutaneously (SC)
3. Magnesium sulfate 2 g by slow IV push (1 minute)
4. Magnesium sulfate 4 g intravenous infusion over 20 minutes.
5. Nitroglycerin for acute intrapartal tocolysis per institutional protocol

NOTE: A protocol for the management of preterm labor that describes the use of tocolytics for patients meeting the criteria for the diagnosis of preterm labor can be found in Appendix D.

Antepartum Monitoring

Evaluation of fetal well-being and maturity is essential in the management of high-risk pregnancy. Generally, routine fetal surveillance through antepartum monitoring and testing is initiated in the event of a nonreassuring sign or when indicated by the high-risk problem (ACOG, 1999c). Gestational age parameters to begin fetal surveillance vary by indication and are initiated when the fetus has a gestational age compatible with life.

This chapter provides information on biophysical assessment (including ultrasound, the biophysical profile, and daily fetal movement count) and on biochemical assessment (including amniocentesis, percutaneous umbilical blood sampling, and chorionic villus sampling). The procedures for nonstress and contraction stress testing and an overview of other fetal assessment parameters are reviewed as well.

Ultrasound

Ultrasound has many uses in obstetrics. There are three levels of ultrasound in obstetrics. They are limited, basic, and comprehensive (ACOG, 1993). The *limited* examination is used for the following: assessment of amniotic fluid volume, biophysical profile parameters, identification of fetal cardiac activity, location of placenta, confirmation of fetal presentation, and certain procedures such as amniocentesis and external cephalic version. The *basic* examination is the most common ultrasound during pregnancy and includes: fetal number, presentation, documentation of cardiac activity, placental location, amniotic fluid volume, assessment of gestational age based on standardized fetal biometries, anatomical survey of the fetus for malformations, and evaluation of the maternal adnexa. If any abnormalities are suspected on previous examination or there is a suspected abnormality based on history or physical examination, the patient is then referred to an examiner with expertise in *comprehensive* ultrasound, usually a perinatologist. Recent guidelines for the use of limited ultrasound by nurses have been developed by the Association of Women's Health, Obstetric and Neonatal Nurses (AWHONN) (Fresquez, 1996). This section presents a short background of ultrasound and its biophysical principles, as well as examples of ultrasound uses.

Background

Experiments using high-frequency sound waves date back to the 1880s, but it was not until World War I that principles of ultrasound were applied to naval science. Most of us are familiar with the term *sonar* (sound navigation and ranging), which refers to the use of high-frequency sound or ultrasound from a ship on the water's surface to detect submerged submarines. The sonar operator of a surface ship would direct a beam of sound into the depths. Upon striking the submerged submarine an echo would return to the sonar source. Based on the time it took for the echo to return after the original sound left the instrument, the operator could calculate the distance and location of that submarine.

Another use of ultrasound that developed during the wartime years was in the detection of flaws in metals used for industrial purposes.

The use of ultrasound in medicine was first reported in the late 1940s in the detection of cranial abnormalities, intracranial tumors, and gallstones. Technological advances in the last 20 years have made ultrasound diagnosis and evaluation easily available and a principal tool used in obstetrics and gynecology.

Biophysical Principles

Ultrasound is the use of those sound waves beyond the range of human hearing. Sound is measured in hertz (Hz), which denotes cycles per second. The frequency range of human hearing is from 20 to 20,000 Hz. The frequency range used in diagnostic ultrasound is 2 to 10 mega (million) hertz (MHz) and is determined by the transducer, which converts electrical energy into sound waves. The transducer contains crystals or elements that have piezoelectric properties. The word *piezoelectric* is derived from the German language and literally translates as "pressure electric." Crystalline quartz, lithium sulfate, lead zirconate, and barium titanate have piezoelectric properties—the ability to convert mechanical pressure into electrical energy and vice versa. The crystal is struck electrically to produce a mechanical pulse. When ultrasound produced by the crystal transverses an object at a 90-degree angle, or is perpendicular to it, the echoes returning to the crystal probe are recorded as dots of light on a cathode ray oscilloscope screen. The intensity and brightness of the dots correspond to the density and acoustic impedance or resistance met by the searching beam of sound at the various tissue interfaces. By moving the transducer in a specific scanning motion, the echoes from each tissue interface coalesce to trace the anatomical outline of that region. Instrumentation technology has improved significantly over the last decade. The ultrasound transducer most commonly used in the obstetrical/gynecological setting is a curved linear array real-time transducer with a frequency of 3.5 to 7.0 MHz. This produces images faster than the eye can perceive so that the image appears to be in real time. Choosing the frequency of the transducer to use depends on the depth that must be penetrated. The faster the frequency, the shallower is the depth of penetration but the better is the resolution of the received echoes. In most term or near-term pregnancies, 3.5 MHz is necessary to visualize the entire uterine depth. The following list contrasts sound frequency with various descriptive uses.

audible range
      20 Hz
      60 Hz Boom of a bass drum
      84 Hz Bass voice
   256 Hz Middle C on piano
 1125 Hz Soprano voice
20,000 Hz

inaudible
 50,000 Hz Ultrasonic cleaners

diagnostic ultrasound
 1,000,000 Hz
 3,500,000 Hz Obstetrical diagnosis
15,000,000 Hz

Safety

A safe level of ultrasound intensity has been defined, and most diagnostic ultrasound instruments produce energies far below that level. Ultrasound exposures at these intensities have not been found to cause any harmful biological effects on patients, fetuses, or instrument operators in over 30 years of research. However, because there is a potential for future identification of risks it is recommended that ultrasound be used prudently and only when there is an indication (AIUM, 1998).

Examples of Ultrasonography

Usually an abdominal and pelvic examination can determine fetal lie. In an obese patient or one who is difficult to examine it is sometimes impossible to determine whether the fetus is in a breech or vertex presentation or a transverse lie. Ultrasound examination can readily determine fetal presentation (Figures 8-1 through 8-6).

Indications for Ultrasound

The indications for ultrasound during pregnancy are as follows (ACOG, 1993):

Estimation of gestational age for patients with uncertain dates or verification of dates for those who will have elective termination or delivery of pregnancy

Evaluation of fetal growth

Vaginal bleeding in pregnancy

Suspected ectopic pregnancy

Identification of multiple gestation (Figure 8-7)

Diagnosis of molar pregnancy

Detection of certain fetal abnormalities

Detection of hydramnios and oligohydramnios

Diagnosis of fetal death

Suspected abruption

Confirmation of fetal lie, position, and presenting part

Guidance for amniocentesis

Biophysical evaluation

Amniotic fluid index

Observation of intrapartum events

Abnormal triple marker screen

Estimation of fetal weight in preterm labor

Follow-up evaluation of identified problem

History of previous fetal anomaly

Evaluation of late registrants for prenatal care

Text continued on p. 164

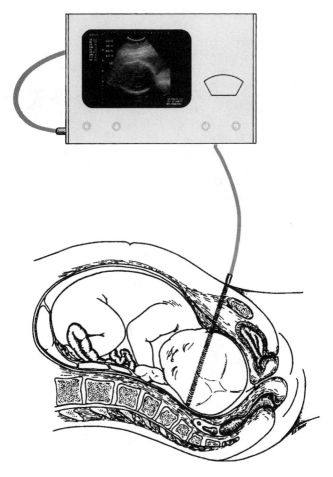

Figure 8-1
The fetal head is displayed on the screen when the
ultrasound transducer is perpendicular to fetal biparietal
diameter (BPD). The BPD is determined by measuring
distance between proximal and distal skull echoes.

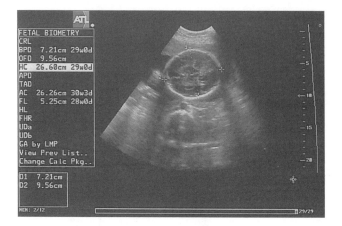

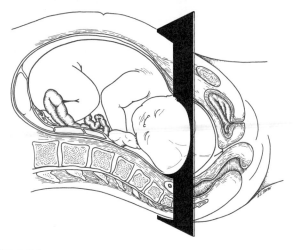

Figure 8-2
Schema of transverse section illustrates fetal head in
sonogram.

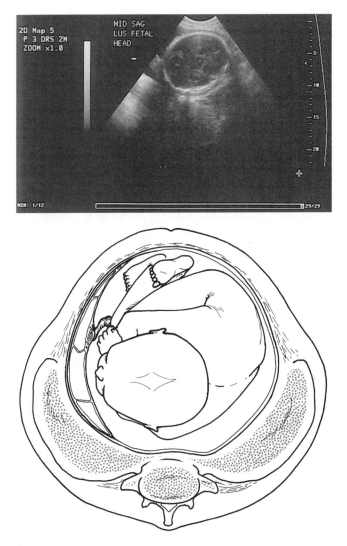

Figure 8-3
Sonogram contrasted with schema of cephalic presentation
in transverse section.

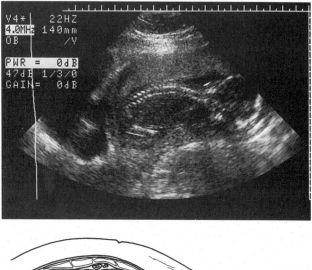

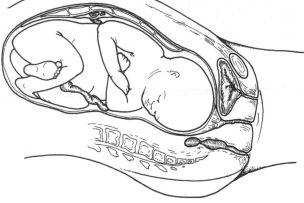

Figure 8-4
Sonogram contrasted with schema of cephalic presentation
in *longitudinal section.*

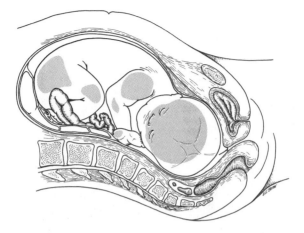

Figure 8-5
Schema of longitudinal section illustrates fetal head, body, and extremity in sonogram.

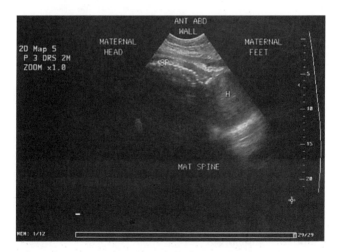

Figure 8-6
Longitudinal view of fetus with head toward maternal feet.

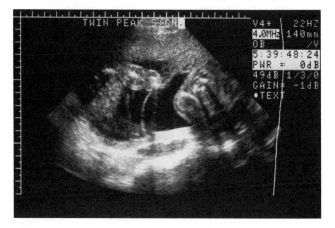

Figure 8-7
Transverse ultrasound of twin gestation. Note membrane
separating amniotic sacs.

Biophysical Profile

Description

The biophysical profile (BPP) is a noninvasive, dynamic assessment of the fetus and fetal environment. The assessment is performed using real-time ultrasound and the electronic fetal heart rate (FHR) monitor. Parameters measured in this evaluation include:

1. Fetal breathing movements (FBM)
2. Fetal movement (FM)
3. Fetal tone (FT)*
4. Amniotic fluid index (AFI)*
5. Non-Stress Test (NST)*

Clinical Significance

FHR reactivity, fetal movements, fetal breathing movements (Figure 8-8), and fetal tone are acute biophysical markers and are be-

---

*Most indicative of fetal well-being.

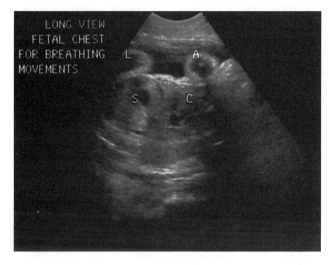

Figure 8-8
Correct view for observing fetal breathing. *A,* Arm; *L,* leg;
S, stomach; *C,* chest.

lieved to be initiated and regulated by complex, integrated mechanisms of the fetal central nervous system. Normal biophysical
activity is indirect evidence that the portion of the central nervous
system that controls that specific activity is intact. However, the
absence of biophysical activities is difficult to interpret because it
may reflect pathological depression or normal fetal periodicity.

The measurement of the amniotic fluid index (AFI) is a marker
of chronic fetal condition.

Investigators have shown an inverse relationship between NST
and AFI findings. The lower the AFI, the greater the incidence of
nonreactive tests, decelerations, and perinatal morbidity and
mortality.

Therefore since the development of the four-quadrant AFI measurement, this technique and the NST, known as the modified BPP,
have been used together with increasing frequency to evaluate both
chronic (AFI) and acute (NST) markers of fetal well-being.

Interpretation

Biophysical profile (BPP) scoring

Biophysical Variable	Normal (Score = 2)	Abnormal (Score = 0)
Fetal breathing movements (FBM)	At least one episode of FBM of at least 30 sec duration in 20-min observation	Absent FBM or <30 sec of sustained FBM in 20 min
Fetal movements (FM)	At least three discrete body/limb movements in 20 min (episodes of active continuous movement considered as a single movement)	Two or fewer episodes of body/limb movements in 20 min
Fetal tone (FT)	At least one episode of active extension with return to flexion of fetal limb(s) or trunk; opening and closing of hand considered normal tone	Either slow extension with return to partial flexion or movement of limb in full extension or absence of fetal movement
Amniotic fluid index (AFI) (varies by gestational age)	Sum total of measurements in cm from each quadrant is 5.1 to 24 cm (low normal is 5.1 to 9.9 cm)	Sum total of measurements in cm from each quadrant is ≤5 cm or >24 cm
Non-Stress Test (NST)	Reactive—two or more episodes of FHR acceleration ≥15 bpm ≥15 sec	Nonreactive

The Biophysical Profile should be recorded on the patient's progress sheet. An example of a BPP scoring format follows:

BPP scoring format

Parameter	Score
Fetal Breathing Movements (FBM)	
Fetal Movement (FM)	
Fetal Tone (FT)	
Amniotic Fluid Index (AFI)	
Non-Stress Test (NST)	
	TOTAL: _____

Management

Guidelines for patient care management based on the BPP score are as follows:

Score	Action
10	Repeat weekly; indicates fetus at minimal risk for fetal damage or death within 1 wk; repeat twice weekly if >42 weeks' gestation or diabetic
8	Repeat weekly; consider delivery if oligohydramnios present; repeat twice weekly if >42 weeks' gestation or diabetic
6	Consider delivery if fetus mature or if oligohydramnios present; if fetus is immature, repeat BPP in 24 hr
4	Deliver unless very immature; repeat within 24 hr
2	Deliver; score has been associated with a perinatal mortality rate of 60% or greater (Gegor, Paine, 1992)

Amniotic Fluid Index Measurement

Procedure	Rationale
Assist patient into the low semi-Fowler's position	To avoid hypotension
	To have enough exposure of the abdomen for placement of ultrasound transducer on the appropriate area of the abdomen
Divide the uterus into four equal quadrants. At term, using the umbilicus, draw an imaginary line across the vertical axis, and using the linea negra, draw an imaginary longitudinal line up and down the abdomen	To divide abdomen into four equal quadrants
Holding the ultrasound transducer in the longitudinal plane and perpendicular to the floor, view each quadrant separately. Using calipers, measure the deepest pocket of fluid in each quadrant. Exclude umbilical cord and fetal parts from measurements	By appropriate placement of the transducer, measuring fluid from an adjacent quadrant is avoided. In addition, keeping the transducer perpendicular avoids an oblique measurement of the pockets, which would result in a falsely increased apparent size of the pocket (Figure 8-9).
Add all values obtained (Figure 8-10)	To determine the amniotic fluid index

Amniotic Fluid Index Values

>24 cm	Increased
10 to 24 cm	Normal
5.1 to 9.9 cm	Low Normal
≤5 cm	Decreased

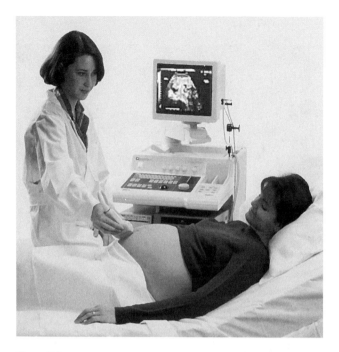

Figure 8-9
Nurse performing amniotic fluid index (AFI) measurement
with the Aloka 650CL ultrasound.
(Courtesy GE Marquette Medical Systems, Milwaukee, Wis.)

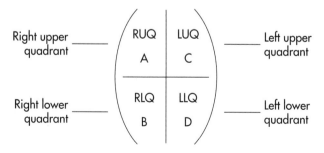

| Right upper quadrant ___ | RUQ
A | LUQ
C | ___ Left upper quadrant |
| Right lower quadrant ___ | RLQ
B | LLQ
D | ___ Left lower quadrant |

Quadrants of the maternal abdomen

Figure 8-10
Amniotic fluid index: AFI is calculated by adding the largest
vertical pocket of amniotic fluid in the four quadrants of the
gravid uterus.   *Continued*

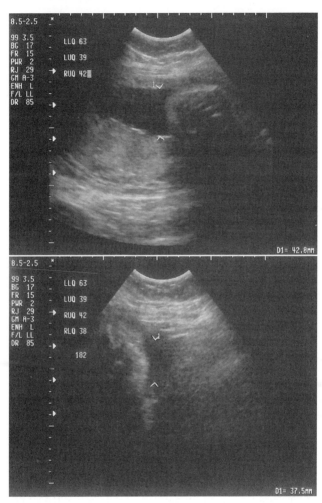

Figure 8-10, cont'd
A, Right upper quadrant (42 mm). **B,** Right lower quadrant
(38 mm).   *Continued*

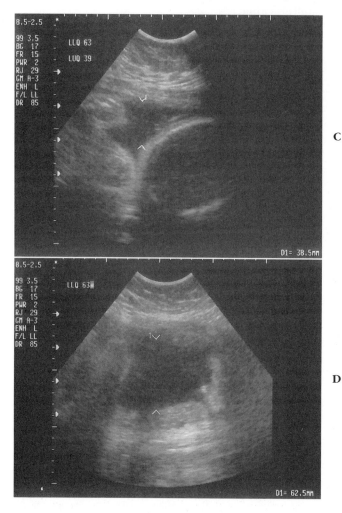

Figure 8-10, cont'd
C, Left upper quadrant (39 mm). **D,** Left lower quadrant
(63 mm). The sum total of amniotic fluid from each of the
four quadrants of this patient was 182 mm (18.2 cm), which
is in the normal range.

Interpretation
Increased AFI (>24 cm)

Increased AFI is an indication for antepartum testing, including se-
rial AFI measurements at least weekly. A complete ultrasound examination should be conducted to evaluate for associated fetal and
placental anomalies, as well as for workup of polyhydramnios, including infection, diabetes, and isoimmunization.

Normal amniotic fluid index (10 to 24 cm)

Normal AFI is a reassuring finding during fetal testing.

Low normal amniotic fluid index (5.1 to 9.9 cm)

Low normal AFI should be evaluated taking into consideration the
gestational age of the fetus. Because amniotic fluid volume peaks
at 34 to 35 weeks' gestation, an AFI of less than 10 cm should be
reevaluated by additional measurements for the presence of associated conditions such as intrauterine growth restriction. A border-
line value of 5.1 cm to 7.0 cm should be reevaluated every 3 to 4
days if all other findings remain normal.

Decreased amniotic fluid index (≤5 cm)

Decreased AFI values of 5 cm or less in a patient at term or post-
term indicate the need to deliver the fetus. When no amniotic fluid
is found, a complete ultrasound examination should be conducted
to rule out fetal anomalies. Rupture of the membranes may be a
cause for decreased or absent amniotic fluid.

Fetal Movement

The number of fetal movements decreases from early to late
pregnancy in normal gestation. In pregnancies complicated by
uteroplacental insufficiency, there is a marked decrease in daily
fetal movement count (DFMC), and a precipitous fall occurs
in the period immediately preceding fetal death. The advantages
of fetal movement counting are that it is inexpensive, continuously available away from the clinical area, and relatively simple
for the patient to do, although accuracy and reliability are
variable.

Parameters for normal daily fetal movement counts or "kick
counts," vary slightly in practice from 3 to 10 movements in 1

hour to 3 in 30 minutes. Procedure varies with time of day, reference to mealtime (just after eating), maternal position (lateral), and hydration (water or juice). The patient is instructed to "be quiet with herself," be relaxed but awake, have an empty bladder, place her hands on her abdomen, and focus on the baby's movements. When the patient is instructed to do kick counts, it is often helpful to use palpation and verify with the patient what sensations can be interpreted as fetal movements. Patients should continue to be aware of fetal movements and report the hourly observations if she perceives decreased fetal movement. It is important to note that fetal movement can occur without maternal recognition (based on studies that show maternal perception is only 40% of actual fetal movement at term [Stanco, 1993]). An NST is often performed if only one or two movements are felt within a 1-hour period. Amniotic fluid indexing may also be done. If the NST is reactive, further testing may not be done unless there are some other risk factors or if the patient again perceives a decrease in fetal movement. A nonreactive NST would be followed as soon as possible by a biophysical profile (BPP) or contraction stress test (CST).

Kick Count Methodology

Patient instructions

Six steps: how to use your counting log

1. Count movements anytime between 7:00 PM and 11:00 PM.
2. After you eat, lie down on your left or right side.
3. Mark down the **date** and **start time** on your log.
4. Place your hands over your abdomen and pay close attention to your baby's movements.
5. Every time your baby moves **or** kicks mark one of the boxes.
6. When the baby has moved **or** kicked 10 times write down the **stop time** on your log.

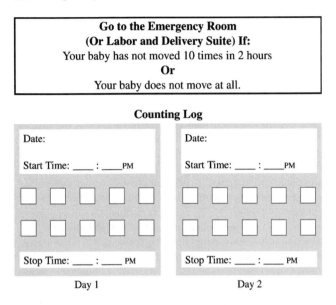

> ## Go to the Emergency Room
> ## (Or Labor and Delivery Suite) If:
> Your baby has not moved 10 times in 2 hours
> ### Or
> Your baby does not move at all.

Counting Log

Date:	Date:
Start Time: ____ : ____PM	Start Time: ____ : ____PM
□ □ □ □ □	□ □ □ □ □
□ □ □ □ □	□ □ □ □ □
Stop Time: ____ : ____ PM	Stop Time: ____ : ____ PM
Day 1	Day 2

Developed by the Women's Hospital Antepartum Testing Unit LAC-USC Medical Center, Los Angeles, Calif. Courtesy Yolanda Rabello, RNC, MS Ed, CCRN.

Umbilical Artery Doppler Velocimetry

Umbilical artery Doppler flow velocimetry is a noninvasive technique used to assess the hemodynamics of vascular impedance. A high-velocity umbilical artery diastolic flow is typically found in normally growing fetuses, whereas diminished flow is found in intrauterine growth-restricted fetuses. The flow can be absent or even reversed in some cases of extreme intrauterine growth restriction. Abnormal flow velocity waveforms have been correlated with fetal hypoxia and acidosis and high perinatal morbidity and mortality. The flow indices generally measured are the systolic to diastolic ratio, resistance index, and pulsatility index. An abnormal flow is either an absent end diastolic flow or a flow index greater than 2 standard deviations above the mean for gestational age. Surveillance of suspected intrauterine growth restriction with umbilical artery Doppler velocimetry can achieve equivalent fetal and neonatal outcomes as primary antepartum surveillance based on the Non-Stress Test (ACOG, 1999c).

Fetoscopy

Fetoscopy is the direct visualization of the fetus with an endoscope inserted into the amniotic cavity through the maternal abdomen. The procedure is done to directly view portions of the fetal anatomy in patients whose fetuses are at high risk for specifically suspected abnormalities and for Ellis–van Creveld syndrome, an autosomal recessive trait in which affected infants have short limbs and cardiac abnormalities and always exhibit polydactyly. This technique has also been used for directing skin biopsies and less frequently to obtain fetal blood in the diagnosis of fetal hemoglobinopathies. Fetoscopy may be used as an adjunct to laser ablation of connecting vessels in twin-twin transfusion syndrome. Real-time ultrasound is used during the procedure to guide the fetoscope to an appropriate area for viewing or blood sampling.

Fetoscopy is generally performed at 18 weeks' gestation. Complications of this procedure are spontaneous abortion, preterm delivery, leakage of amniotic fluid, amnionitis, and intrauterine fetal death.

An analgesic may be given to the patient to limit fetal movement during the procedure. Postprocedure care includes monitoring of vital signs, administration of anti-Rh globulin as indicated, and teaching patients to report any pain, bleeding, amniotic fluid loss, or fever.

Amnioscopy

Amnioscopy is the direct visualization of amniotic fluid through the fetal membranes with a cone-shaped hollow tube when the cervix is sufficiently dilated. It is done to identify meconium staining of the amniotic fluid, which results from an episode of fetal hypoxia causing relaxation of the anal sphincter and an increase in fetal peristalsis.

Amnioscopy is of value in postdate pregnancies when the possibility of postmature syndrome exists.

The amnioscope is also used to visualize the presenting part after rupture of membranes to obtain a fetal blood sample for blood gas analysis. The procedure is performed with the patient in lithotomy position and takes approximately 10 minutes. The patient should be instructed that dilation of the cervix from the endoscope may cause some discomfort and menstrual-type cramping may continue for some time after the procedure is completed. This procedure is rarely done.

Amniography

Amniography is the injection of radiopaque agents into the amniotic sac to identify hydramnios, oligohydramnios, placenta previa, the soft tissue silhouette of the fetus, and—after a few hours of swallowing—the fetal gastrointestinal tract. Meconium staining of the amniotic fluid may follow this procedure, especially if the fetus is approaching term. However, this is not specifically indicative of fetal distress. Because ultrasonography provides most of the information that amniography does without the use of ionizing radiation or injection into the amniotic sac, amniography is rarely done.

Magnetic Resonance Imaging

Magnetic resonance imaging (MRI) is a noninvasive tool that provides excellent visualization of soft tissue. This technique can be used to evaluate fetal structures, placenta position and density, amniotic fluid quantity, maternal structures and soft tissue, and metabolic or functional malformations. The time required for the procedure is rather lengthy, from 20 to 60 minutes, during which the patient must be very still. Although the information gleaned from this procedure is very specific, broad usage is limited because of the time involved, fetal movement, and other acceptable alternatives to obtain similar information.

Computed Tomography

Computed tomography (CT scan) pelvimetry is used occasionally to assess the anatomical pelvis in anticipation of a vaginal breech delivery.

Radiography

Radiological assessment for fetal size and maturity and placental localization is seldom done since the advent of ultrasound diagnosis. In recent years there has been growing concern over the use of ionizing radiation because of potential carcinogenic, teratogenic, and mutagenic effects. The scope of these risks has yet to be clearly identified.

A simple radiograph of the abdomen and pelvis after 16 weeks' gestation will most often identify fetal skeletal parts. During the second half of pregnancy the number of fetuses can be seen in a multiple gestation. Anencephaly and hydrocephaly can be identified during the third trimester. There is some correlation between fetal age and the time of appearance of lower limb ossification centers, but this varies with fetal sex and weight.

Radiography is essentially only done in nonobstetrical applications such as for an intravenous pyelogram (IVP) or trauma, because ultrasound can provide the necessary information regarding the fetus.

Amniocentesis

Amniocentesis, the removal of fluid from the amniotic cavity by needle puncture (Figure 8-11), was described in the early 1950s by Bevis (1952), who noted the varying degrees of bile pigments in amniotic fluid discovered while assessing Rh-isoimmunized pregnancies. Since then, the use of amniocentesis has become a standard tool in the assessment of fetal well-being and maturity and in the diagnosis of genetic defects.

An amniocentesis is the penetration of the amniotic cavity through the abdominal and uterine walls for the purpose of withdrawing fluid for examination. The procedure is performed under ultrasound guidance by insertion of a 20- to 22-gauge spiral-type needle transabdominally to aspirate 5 to 20 ml of amniotic fluid.

When genetic problems are suspected, amniocentesis is performed as soon as possible, usually between 16 and 20 weeks' gestation, to allow for karyotyping and biochemical studies to be completed before the time limit for having an elective termination of pregnancy. If this is not an option for the parents, an amniocentesis may still be advised for pregnancy management considerations and so that the family might prepare for the special needs of a chromosomally abnormal infant.

Amniocentesis later in pregnancy is most often performed to assess fetal well-being and maturity. In cases of isoimmunization the procedure may be performed repeatedly to monitor the fetal condition. In high-risk pregnancies, such as those with maternal diabetes, amniocentesis may be performed to assess fetal lung maturity, indicating the most opportune time for delivery (ACOG, 1996).

There are minimal risks to amniocentesis. Several researchers have reported that fewer than 0.5% of all amniocentesis procedures result in spontaneous abortion. Other risks include trauma to the fetus or to the placenta, bleeding, infection, premature labor, and

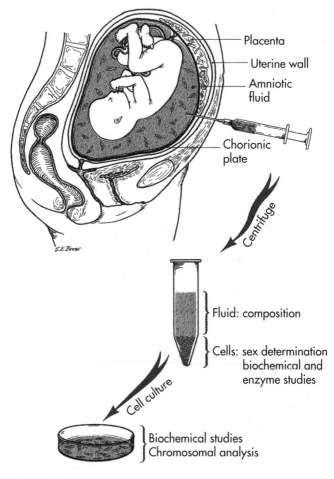

Figure 8-11
Amniocentesis. Amniotic fluid is aspirated with a sterile
syringe. Sample is centrifuged to separate cells and fluid.
A variety of tests can be done.

Rh sensitization from fetal bleeding into the maternal circulation. Overall, however, the risk of amniocentesis to the mother or the fetus is generally accepted to be in the range of 0.5%. This is markedly reduced partially because of the use of ultrasonographic guidance during the procedure.

Before amniocentesis for any reason the physician informs the patient of specific risk factors. This verbal interaction is documented by a consent form. Although the wording varies from institution to institution, the forms are consistent in basic content. They include the following key points:

1. The risk factor to mother and fetus is approximately 0.5%.
2. The culture of fetal cells may not be successful.
3. Repeated amniocentesis may be required.
4. Chromosome analysis, biochemical analysis, or both may not be successful.
5. Normal chromosome results, normal biochemical results, or both do not eliminate the possibility that the child may have birth defects or mental retardation because of other disorders.

Patient Care

The nurse has a key role in supporting the patient through the procedure of amniocentesis because patients approach it with a variety of feelings and questions. Initially the patient may wonder whether she should expose herself and her fetus to the risk of amniocentesis. She may use the results to decide if she will terminate an abnormal pregnancy. She may question the ramifications of continuing a pregnancy with an abnormal fetus, projecting her thoughts past delivery into the "quality of life" issue. The nurse can act as a support figure by being knowledgeable about the procedure, by answering questions factually, and by reinforcing explanations given by the physician.

During amniocentesis the nurse should stand by the side or at the head of the patient. The patient must remain quiet during the procedure and must be instructed not to touch the abdomen or drapes. Placing the patient's hands under her head serves as a reminder. Because most women are quite anxious when they see the length of the needle, they should be visually distracted or requested to close their eyes before needle entry. Patients who do not watch needle insertion usually report feeling only a sense of pressure on the abdomen.

Body proximity, eye contact, and touch by the nurse offer a sense of security and support. A damp washcloth on a perspiring forehead may be soothing. A nervous hand held by the nurse may be comforting. Anxious words and impromptu comments should be accepted by the nurse with a supportive attitude.

When the amniocentesis is completed, the patient should be observed for any untoward symptoms. If the patient feels faint, she should be assisted in turning to her left side. This will counteract any *supine hypotension* (caused by uterine pressure on the vena cava) by increasing venous return, blood pressure, and cardiac output. The patient's vital signs should be monitored postprocedure. The uterine fundus should be palpated at the same time to note fetal or uterine activity.

When the patient has fully recovered, she should be instructed to report any of the following to the physician: vaginal drainage, uterine contractions, signs of infection such as fever or chills, abdominal pain, and vaginal bleeding.

Amniotic Fluid Analysis

Amniotic fluid derives mostly from fetal urine and secretions and contains fetal cells. The sample is centrifuged to separate the cells from the fluid.

Color

A bloody tap may result in cell growth failure and changes the level of other amniotic fluid constituents in the direction of predicting a less mature fetus.

A greenish-tinged or a thick, dark-green sample indicates the presence of meconium. Aside from indicating a patent fetal anus, the presence of meconium is generally accepted to be associated with some degree of fetal hypoxia. However, the exact cause for the presence of meconium is not known, and it is often observed in the absence of hypoxia. The presence of meconium interferes with the reliability of other tests such as the L/S ratio and the bilirubin ΔOD.

Lecithin/sphingomyelin (L/S) ratio

Pulmonary surfactant primarily contains phospholipids. Surfactant acts as a surface detergent at the air-liquid interface of the alveoli, preventing their collapse at the end of an expiration. Without surfactant a neonate develops respiratory distress syndrome (RDS), a condition associated with immaturity in which the alveoli of the lung literally collapse with each expiration.

The L/S ratio assesses two phospholipids—lecithin and sphingomyelin—that compose the largest part of the surfactant complex. Normally during gestation the sphingomyelin concentrations are greater than those of lecithin until about 26 weeks' gestation. From 26 to 33 weeks' gestation the concentration of lecithin to sphingomyelin is fairly equal, and therefore the L/S ratio is approximately 1 : 1. From 34 to 36 weeks' gestation there is a sudden increase in lecithin and the ratio rapidly rises. It is generally accepted that a ratio of 2.0 or greater indicates pulmonary maturity and that respiratory distress syndrome (RDS) will rarely occur in the neonate. In a macrosomic fetus, as occurs in a diabetic gestation, the association between the L/S ratio and RDS is adversely affected. (See following discussion of Lung Profile.) The following interpretation is generally accepted:

L/S Ratio	Fetal Lung	Risk for RDS
>2.0	Mature	Minimal
1.50 to 2.0	Transitional zone	Moderate
<1.50	Immature	High

Some stressful conditions during pregnancy have been known to accelerate fetal lung maturity. They include preeclampsia, prolonged ruptured membranes, narcotic addiction, and intrauterine growth retardation. This acceleration may be a reflex fetal response to a hostile intrauterine environment. In contrast, conditions in which fetal lung maturity tends to be delayed include diabetes mellitus and fetal hemolytic disease.

Acceleration of fetal lung maturity can be achieved when the glucocorticoid betamethasone is injected into patients in whom premature delivery is anticipated. The fetal lung matures, as reflected by a rise in the L/S ratio usually within 48 hours after initiating therapy.

The technique used to measure the L/S ratio by thin-layer chromatography was developed by Gluck and associates (Gluck, 1971). To reduce laboratory time in performing the L/S ratio, the foam stability or "shake test" was introduced by Clements (1972) and co-workers. The "shake test" is based on the ability of surfactant to generate a stable foam when ethanol is added to the amni-

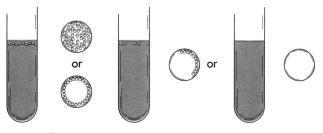

Positive foam test   Negative foam test

Figure 8-12
Clement's foam test (the shake test). For test to be positive, bubbles must be seen around entire circumference of tube.

otic fluid specimen. Ethanol, isotonic saline, and amniotic fluid in measured amounts and varying dilutions are shaken together for 15 seconds. A ring of bubbles at the air-liquid interface at the proper dilution after 15 minutes indicates probable fetal lung maturity (Figure 8-12).

Measurement of the L/S ratio may be omitted when the "shake test" is positive because false-positive tests are rare. False-negative tests, however, are common and require awaiting the L/S ratio. The shake test is infrequently used today because more accurate results can be obtained with the L/S ratio.

Lung profile

The association between the L/S ratio and the incidence of respiratory distress syndrome does not always hold true in the diabetic gestation. RDS has been reported in neonates who had mature L/S ratios. The Lung Profile overcomes the problem of assessing lung maturity in the fetus of the diabetic and adds a parameter of security when interruption of pregnancy is contemplated.

The Lung Profile measures the interrelationships among the surfactant phospholipids: the lecithin/sphingomyelin (L/S) ratio, disaturated (acetone precipitated) lecithin (PL), phosphatidyl inositol (PI), and phosphatidyl glycerol (PG). Functional maturity of the lung occurs with the combination of these phospholipids. Phosphatidyl glycerol acts as a lung stabilizer, and when it is present in diabetic gestations with a mature L/S ratio, one can be confident that RDS will not occur.

Table 8-1   Various biochemical monitoring techniques*

Test	Results	Significance of Findings
Maternal Blood		
Triple marker screening†		
Serum alpha-fetoprotein (AFP)	Low level	Possible Down syndrome
β-hCG	High level	
Unconjugated estriol (E₃)	Low level	
Human placental lactogen	High levels	Large diabetic fetus; multiple gestation
	Low levels	Threatened abortion; IUGR; postmaturity
Alpha-fetoprotein	>40 ng/ml	Fetal neural tube defect
Coombs' test	Titer of 1:8 and rising	Significant isoimmunization
Amniocentesis		
Color	Meconium	Possible hypoxia
Lung Profile		Fetal lung maturity
L/S ratio	≥2.0	
PL	>50%	

*In an effort to summarize these studies in tabular form, generalizations have been made.
†From Benn et al, 1995 and Mooney et al, 1994.
IUGR, Intrauterine growth restriction; *L/S,* lecithin/sphingomyelin ratio; *PI,* phosphatidyl inositol; *PG,* phosphatidyl glycerol; *PL,* disaturated (acetone precipitated) lecithin. *Continued*

Table 8-1   Various biochemical monitoring techniques—cont'd

Test	Results	Significance of Findings
Amniocentesis—cont'd		
Lung Profile—cont'd		
PI	15%-20%	
PG	2%-10%	
Amniostat	PG ≥2 µg/ml	Fetal lung maturity
Disaturated phosphatidylcholine (DSPC)	≥500 µg/dL	Fetal lung maturity
Shake test	Complete ring of bubbles after shaking at 1:2 dilution	Fetal lung maturity
Foam stability index	≥47	Fetal lung maturity
Lamellar body count	>30,000	Fetal lung maturity
Bilirubin (ΔOD 450) (Figure 8-13)	<0.015	Gestational age >36 wk; normal pregnancy
	High levels	Fetal hemolytic disease in isoimmunized pregnancies
Lipid cells	>10%	Gestational age >35 wk
Alpha-fetoprotein	High levels after 15 wk gestation	Open neural tube defect
Osmolality	Decline after 20 wk gestation	Advancing nonspecific gestational age
Genetic disorders Sex-linked Chromosomal Metabolic	Dependent on cultured cells for karyotype and enzymatic activity	

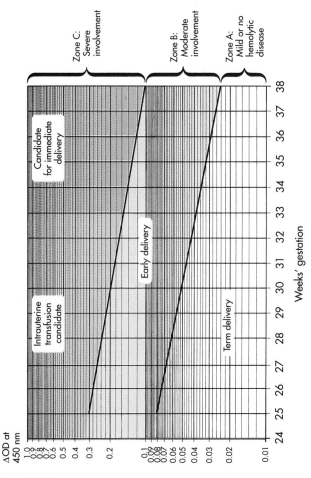

Figure 8-13
Prediction of severity of fetal hemolytic disease from
amniotic fluid bilirubin with management guidelines.

Amniostat-FLM is an immunologic test with agglutination in the presence of phosphatidyl glycerol indicating lung maturity.

Amniotic fluid bilirubin

During the second half of pregnancy the concentration of amniotic fluid bilirubin decreases until it virtually disappears during the last month of gestation. This measurement can be used to complement other laboratory values in assessing gestational age. However, it is not sensitive enough to be used alone for that purpose and has generally been replaced by the L/S ratio.

Amniotic fluid bilirubin is usually analyzed with a spectrophotometer measuring the optical density (OD) of the specimen against the characteristic absorption peak at 450 nm.* The value is usually expressed as ΔOD 450. It is important that the specimen of amniotic fluid not be exposed to light at any time for more than a few seconds, because this can invalidate the test. Amber glass specimen containers can be used, or clear test tubes can be covered with occlusive tape to protect the specimen from light.

In Rh-negative–sensitized pregnancies, as identified by maternal antibody titer (indirect Coombs' test), amniocentesis for bilirubin is one method of evaluating the severity of fetal hemolytic disease (see Figure 8-13).

Percutaneous Umbilical Blood Sampling

Percutaneous umbilical blood sampling is achieved through the transabdominal insertion of a needle into a fetal umbilical vessel under ultrasound guidance. The ideal insertion point is near the placental insertion. Between 1 and 4 ml of blood are removed during the procedure and tested by the Kleihauer-Betke procedure to ensure that the specimen is fetal blood. The blood sample is used for determining karyotyping, direct Coombs', CBC, fetal blood type, blood gases, acid-base status for intrauterine growth restriction fetuses, detection of infection, and assessment and treatment of isoimmunization.

Complications are unusual and are due to blood leakage from the puncture site, fetal bradycardia, and chorioamnionitis (Bald et al, 1991) (Figure 8-14).

---

*In the Système International d'Unités (SI) nanometer (nm) replaces millimicron (mμ) as the designation for 10^{-9} meters.

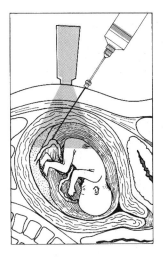

Figure 8-14
Technique for percutaneous umbilical blood sampling guided
by ultrasound.
(From Lowdermilk D, Perry S, Bobak I: *Maternity and women's health care,* ed 7,
St Louis, 2000, Mosby.)

Chorionic Villus Sampling

Chorionic villus sampling (CVS) is the transcervical or transabdominal insertion of a needle into the fetal portion of the placenta
to remove a small tissue specimen. The procedure is done between
10 and 12 weeks' gestation. The procedure is performed under real-
time ultrasound visualization. The aspiration cannula and obturator
traverse the cervical canal, and caution is exercised to avoid rupturing the amniotic sac. A transabdominal approach is an alternative
to the transcervical technique. This procedure can be performed
early in the first trimester to identify fetuses with genetic defects.
Complications are rare after the procedure and include vaginal spot-
ting or bleeding, spontaneous abortion, rupture of membranes, and
chorioamnionitis. Rh immune globulin should be given to Rh-
negative women because of the possibility of fetomaternal hemorrhage, which could result in isoimmunization (Figure 8-15).

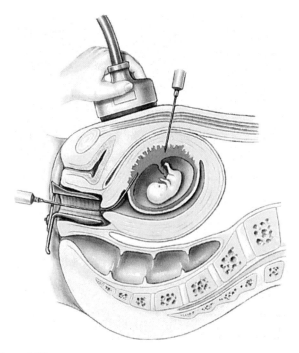

Figure 8-15
Chorionic villi sampling. Taking sample by transcervical method.
(Courtesy Medical and Scientific Illustration, Crozet, Va.)

Non-Stress and Stress Testing

The Contraction Stress Test (CST), the Non-Stress Test (NST), and fetal movement counts have been widely employed for the determination of fetal well-being.

Some indications for both the NST and the CST follow:
1. Suspected postmaturity (postdates ≥41 weeks)
2. Maternal diabetes mellitus
3. Chronic hypertension
4. Hypertensive disorders in pregnancy
5. Suspected and documented IUGR
6. Sickle cell disease
7. Maternal cyanotic heart disease

8. History of previous stillbirth
9. Blood group sensitization (isoimmunization)
10. Meconium-stained amniotic fluid (at amniocentesis)
11. Hyperthyroidism
12. Collagen vascular diseases
13. Older gravida (more than 35 years)
14. Chronic renal disease
15. Decreasing (or apparently absent) fetal movement
16. Severe maternal anemia
17. Discordant twins
18. Multiple gestation
19. High-risk antepartum patients (premature rupture of membranes, preterm labor, and bleeding)

Non-Stress Test

Description

The basis for the NST to assess fetal well-being is that the normal fetus will produce characteristic heart rate patterns. Average baseline variability and acceleration of FHR in response to fetal movement are reassuring signs. The FHR pattern is assessed by external monitoring techniques without any stress or stimuli to the fetus.

When hypoxia, acidosis, or drugs depress the fetal CNS, there may be a reduction in baseline variability and absence of FHR acceleration with fetal movement. The patterns can also be produced by quiet fetal sleep states, and therefore it is sometimes necessary to monitor 20 to 30 minutes or more until the fetus is in a more active state or to palpate the abdomen or use vibroacoustic stimulation (VAS) to activate the resting fetus. The efficacy of maternal ingestion of food or fluids to stimulate the fetus has not been established.

Contraindications

There are no contraindications to the NST.

Preparation and Procedure

An advantage of the NST over the CST is that it can be performed in an outpatient setting. Prepare the patient for the NST by taking a baseline blood pressure, then applying the external mode of monitoring with the patient in semi-Fowler's position and with a lateral tilt (Figure 8-16).

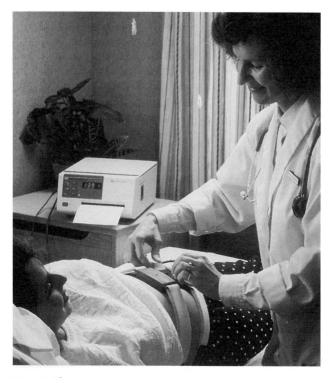

Figure 8-16
Antepartum monitoring.
(Courtesy GE Marquette Medical Systems, Milwaukee, Wis.)

The observer identifies fetal movement on the chart paper as evidenced by spikes or momentary increases in uterine pressure. The new generation of electronic fetal monitors are sensitive to fetal movements and mark their occurrence. If evidence of fetal movement is not apparent on the chart paper, the patient is asked to depress an event button when she perceives fetal movement. The "event" of fetal movement is then noted by a vertical line printed by the stylus on the uterine activity (UA) section of the monitor strip. Fetal monitors with Doppler fetal movement detection capability detect movements automatically and record them simultaneously with FHR and uterine activity. These monitors have been shown to detect gross fetal trunk movements with a very good correlation to such ultrasound detected movements (Melendez, Rayburn, Smith, 1992; Besinger, Johnson, 1989). This capability is important in that fetal movement is not always accurately perceived by the mother. In addition, this FHR-FMP (Fetal Movement Profile) employs two of the five parameters of the Biophysical Profile and its use may prevent the necessity of a Contraction Stress Test (Stanco et al, 1993).

If necessary, fetal movement can be facilitated by palpation of the abdomen or VAS to activate the fetus. If indicated, maternal blood pressure may be monitored during and at the end of the procedure. The procedure usually lasts 20 minutes but may need to be extended if criteria for a reactive pattern have not been met. If the pattern is questionable or if decelerations occur, a Biophysical Profile (BPP) and/or CST may then be performed, or monitoring may be continued until interpretable data are obtained.

Interpretation

The following guidelines for evaluation of the NST are offered, although minor variations in criteria are successfully used by various institutions.

Reactive test (Figure 8-17)	Two or more FHR accelerations above baseline of at least 15 bpm lasting at least 15 seconds in a 20-minute period; baseline rate is within the normal range, and variability is average
Nonreactive test (Figure 8-18)	Absence of accelerations of FHR during the testing period
Inconclusive test	Less than one acceleration above baseline in a 20-minute period or one that is less than 15 bpm and lasts less than 15 seconds; variability less than 6 bpm or quality of FHR recording not adequate for interpretation

Clinical Significance and Management

The reactive test suggests that the fetus will be born in good condition if labor occurs in a few days. However, when the NST is used for primary fetal surveillance, it should be performed twice weekly in high-risk patients, especially those with postdate pregnancies and diabetes or intrauterine growth restriction. As long as twice-weekly NSTs remain reactive, most high-risk pregnancies

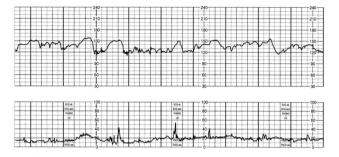

Figure 8-17
Reactive Non-Stress Test (FHR acceleration with fetal movement).

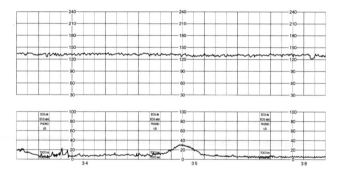

Figure 8-18
Nonreactive Non-Stress Test (no FHR acceleration with fetal movement).

are allowed to continue. The nonreactive test should be followed as soon as possible by a CST. Patients with an inconclusive test may have the NST repeated in several hours or may have a CST or BPP, according to the clinical assessment of the physician.

Inasmuch as a nonreactive or inconclusive test can be caused by fetal sleep states, an attempt should be made to stimulate the fetus by manipulating the uterus or by stimulating the fetus with VAS and continuing to monitor the fetus for another 20- or 30-minute period.

Current trends reported in the literature are to combine NST with amniotic fluid index (AFI) readings of BPP in the fetal surveillance of high-risk pregnancies. Depending on gestational age or deliverability, the nonreactive test should be followed as soon as possible by a BPP and/or CST. Patients with an inconclusive test may have the NST repeated in several hours or may have a BPP and/or CST, according to the clinical assessment of the provider.

Vibroacoustic Stimulation

The vibroacoustic stimulation (VAS) test evaluates the FHR response to acoustic stimulation. Acceleration of FHR with vibro-acoustic stimulation, as well as with fetal movement, is predictive of fetal outcome. This test may also be called a *fetal acoustic stimulation test (FAST)*.

The procedure for this test is as follows:
1. Monitor the FHR and uterine activity until at least 20 minutes of interpretable data are obtained. If there are no spontaneous accelerations of FHR, proceed to the next step.
2. Apply the artificial larynx or a fetal acoustic stimulation device firmly to the maternal abdomen over the fetal head.
3. Depress the button on the device for a single 1- to 2-second sound stimulation. At the same time, it is preferable to depress the event marker, which will mark the uterine activity panel of the monitor strip.
4. Observe and document the FHR response to the stimulation.
5. Repeat the stimulus after 1 minute if there is no acceleration response. An additional repeat with 2 seconds of VAS may be done if necessary.

Interpretation

Reactive test: Two FHR accelerations of 15 bpm above baseline for 15 seconds in response to acoustic stimulation within 20 minutes

Nonreactive test: Inability to fulfill the criterion for reactivity as described above.

Clinical Significance and Management

A reactive test is associated with fetal well-being and suggests that the fetus will be born in good condition if labor occurs within a week. Management beyond that time includes ongoing surveillance. A nonreactive test should be followed by a BPP and/or CST.

There have been reports of fetal tachycardia occurring as a result of VAS and a delay of several minutes to return to baseline. If this occurs, the FHR should continue to be monitored until the FHR returns to baseline.

Contraction Stress Test

The basis for the CST is that a healthy fetus can withstand a decreased oxygen supply during the physiological stress of a contraction, whereas a compromised fetus will demonstrate late decelerations that are nonreassuring and indicative of uteroplacental insufficiency.

CSTs can be performed with endogenously produced oxytocin as stimulated by breast and nipple manipulation, or the test can be performed with an exogenous source of oxytocin administered by IV infusion.

Although the NST can be performed on any patient, the CST cannot. The potential for preterm labor precludes performing the test on patients with certain high-risk conditions and gestational ages.

The CST is contraindicated in the following situations:
1. Premature rupture of membranes
2. Placenta previa
3. Third-trimester bleeding
4. Previous classical cesarean section
5. Multiple gestation
6. Incompetent cervix
7. Hydramnios
8. Risk for preterm delivery

The two types of CST are the nipple-stimulated contraction stress test and the oxytocin challenge test.

Nipple-Stimulated Contraction Stress Test

Procedure	Rationale
1. Assist the patient to a semi-Fowler's position with lateral tilt	1. To avoid supine hypotension
2. Place the tocotransducer where the least maternal tissue is in evidence, usually above the umbilicus	2. To ensure that the fundus is as close as possible to the pressure-sensing device

Procedure	Rationale
3. Place the ultrasound transducer on the maternal abdomen where the clearest fetal signal can be obtained	3. To ensure that the tracing is clear and interpretable
4. Monitor baseline FHR and uterine activity until 10 minutes of interpretable data are obtained (defer nipple stimulation if three spontaneous unstimulated contractions of more than 40-seconds duration occur within a 10-minute period)	4. To provide a basis for comparison (it may not be necessary to proceed with test if spontaneous contractions occur)
5. Instruct patient to brush palmar surface of the fingers over the nipple of one breast through her clothes; continue four cycles of 2 minutes on and 2 to 5 minutes off; stop when contraction begins and restimulate when contraction ends (if a 2-minute period has elapsed)	5. To stimulate oxytocin secretion into the circulation from the pituitary gland
a. If unsuccessful after four cycles, restimulate the breasts for 10 minutes, stopping when contraction begins and resuming when contraction ends	a. To maintain uterine contractions
b. If unsuccessful, begin bilateral continuous stimulation for 10 minutes, stopping when contraction begins and resuming when contraction ends	
6. Discontinue nipple stimulation when three or more spontaneous contractions lasting longer than 40 seconds occur in a 10-minute period and are palpable to the	6. To eliminate unnecessary stress

Procedure	Rationale
examiner. Discontinue the oxytocin if there is evidence of hyperstimulation, prolonged bradycardia, or consistent late decelerations; treat fetal distress in the same manner as during intrapartum monitoring; be prepared to administer terbutaline for tocolysis	
7. Interpret results and continue monitoring until uterine activity has returned to the prestimulation state	7. To ensure that the patient and fetus are restored to their prestress status

If nipple stimulation does not produce the desired uterine activity, an oxytocin-stimulated CST is indicated (Huddleston, 1984). Interpretation guidelines for CST are described after the Oxytocin Challenge Test (OCT).

Oxytocin Challenge Test

The Oxytocin Challenge Test (OCT) is routinely performed in the inpatient setting because labor may be stimulated in some sensitive patients, particularly in those at term.

Procedure	Rationale
1. Assist patient into a semi-Fowler's position with lateral tilt	1. To avoid supine hypotension
2. Place the tocotransducer where the least maternal tissue is in evidence, usually above the umbilicus	2. To ensure that the fundus is as close as possible to the pressure-sensing button
3. Place the ultrasound transducer where the clearest fetal heart sound can be heard, usually below the umbilicus	3. To obtain a clear fetal signal
4. Monitor baseline FHR and uterine activity until 10	4. To provide a basis for comparison

Procedure	Rationale
minutes of interpretable data are obtained before administration of oxytocin	
5. Check the patient's blood pressure and pulse every 10 to 15 minutes	5. To identify hypotension resulting from maternal position
6. If less than three spontaneous unstimulated contractions occur within a 10-minute period and if late decelerations do not occur with spontaneous contractions, oxytocin can be initiated	6. Oxytocin stimulation may not be necessary if adequate uterine activity is present; test may be discontinued if late decelerations occur with spontaneous contractions
7. Piggyback oxytocin into the primary IV line (with lactated Ringer's or other non-aqueous solution) near IV hub	7. May be necessary to stop oxytocin and rapidly infuse the primary IV in the event of uterine hyperstimulation or maternal hypotension
8. Administer oxytocin beginning with 0.5 to 2.0 mU/min with a constant infusion pump per unit protocol	8. To ensure specific dosage of oxytocin
9. Increase the dosage of oxytocin infusion by 0.5 to 1.0 mU/min at 15-minute intervals until the contraction frequency is three in 10 minutes of 40- to 60-seconds duration and contractions are palpable to the examiner	9. To ensure a safe rate of oxytocin increments; generally the dosage of oxytocin does not exceed 5 mU/min, but on rare occasions doses of up to 10 mU/min may be necessary
10. Discontinue the oxytocin when three contractions have occurred within a 10-minute period of interpretable data	10. To provide an adequate stress from which an interpretation can be made
11. Discontinue the oxytocin any time there is evidence of hyperstimulation, pro-	11. To prevent additional fetal distress; the principles for treating fetal distress apply

Procedure	Rationale
longed bradycardia, or consistent late decelerations; treat fetal distress in the same manner as during intrapartum monitoring; be prepared to administer terbutaline for tocolysis	during both antepartum and intrapartum monitoring
12. Continue to monitor until uterine activity and FHR return to baseline status	12. To ensure that the patient and fetus are restored to their prestress status

Interpretation

1. Negative test (Figure 8-19)	1. Three uterine contractions in a 10-minute period without late decelerations; there is usually average baseline variability and acceleration of FHR with fetal movement
2. Positive test (Figure 8-20)	2. Persistent late decelerations or late decelerations with more than half the contractions; may be associated with minimal or absent variability
3. Suspicious test	3. Late decelerations occurring with less than half the uterine contractions

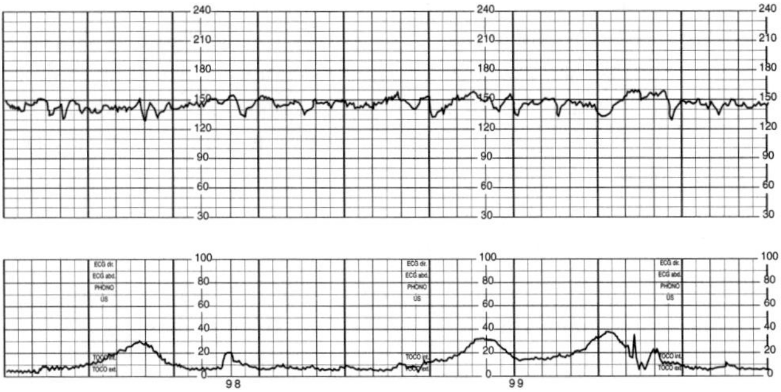

Figure 8-19
Negative Contraction Stress Test (reassuring external tracing).

4. Hyperstimulation

4. Contractions occurring more often than every 2 minutes or lasting longer than 90 seconds, or if there is apparent hypertonus associated with contractions; if no late decelerations occur with the preceding, the test is interpreted as negative; if late deceleration is observed during or after excessive uterine activity, the test is not interpretable and is classified as hyperstimulation because the stress is considered enough to exceed even normal uteroplacental reserve

5. Unsatisfactory

5. Quality of the recording is not sufficient to be sure that no late decelerations are present or where less than three uterine contractions have occurred in a 10-minute period; the test is not interpretable and cannot be used for clinical management

The CST is highly reliable when it is negative. False negatives are rare. On the other hand, false positives can occur if hyperstimulation patterns are unrecognized or if maternal position is supine, resulting in hypotension and late decelerations.

In contrast, when there is an absence of late decelerations in a patient in labor with a previous positive CST, it may be indicative

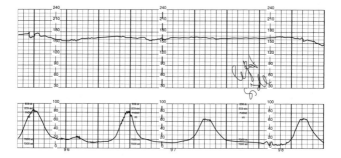

Figure 8-20
Positive Contraction Stress Test (late deceleration with uterine contractions).

of a correction of uteroplacental insufficiency in the interval between the test and labor and not a false positive CST.

Clinical Significance and Management

A negative CST is reassuring that the fetus is likely to survive labor should it occur within 1 week, as long as there is no change in status of either the mother or the fetus. This may permit a postponement of intervention until fetal lung maturity is achieved. As an indicator of fetoplacental respiratory reserve, the CST cannot prevent fetal death from obstetrical emergencies such as abruptio placentae and prolapsed cord. Preterm labor is not associated with a CST. If the fetus is less than 38 weeks' gestation, labor almost never begins within 48 hours after the procedure.

Immediate retesting is required if there is a sudden change in maternal condition of the following: lupus flare, diabetes out of control, sickle cell crisis, worsening preeclampsia/pregnancy-induced hypertension, worsening renal disease, severe maternal dehydration, and an acute asthmatic episode.

The literature reports a false positive rate as high as 30% (Gegor, Paine, 1992). Therefore management of the patient with a positive CST is not clear cut. Fetal assessment utilizing other techniques such as BPP is indicated. In some cases, immediate termination of pregnancy may be warranted.

Home Uterine Activity Monitoring (HUAM) for Patients at Risk for Preterm Labor

Home uterine activity monitoring (HUAM) has been used in an attempt to prevent preterm births. This has been achieved with the utilization of a lightweight tocodynamometer designed for ambulatory home monitoring, data storage, and telephone transmission of uterine activity. Patients using this device have been given detailed instructions regarding the frequency of self-monitoring and asked to phone daily transmissions to a central monitoring unit. An obstetrical nurse interprets the data and then advises the patient as appropriate for the uterine activity noted on the transmission. The patient may be told to take additional tocolytic agents, increase hydration, empty the bladder, be remonitored, and then be referred to a primary care center for further evaluation (Stringer et al, 1994). Some visiting nursing or home health nursing agencies perform home monitoring in conjunction with a home visit. Thus the nurse is present during the monitoring and can perform further physical evaluation (palpation and vaginal examination) if warranted by the assessed uterine activity. Self-palpation by the patient is another method of monitoring uterine activity without a monitor but with daily telephone contact between the patient and a nurse.

In a study (Dyson et al, 1998) conducted between July, 1992 and August, 1996 in women receiving prenatal care at 30 outpatient offices in northern California, 2422 pregnant women with known risk factors for preterm labor were assigned to receive the same type of education and to one of three groups. The groups were:

1. Weekly contact with a nurse
2. Daily contact with a nurse
3. Daily contact with a nurse and home uterine activity monitoring

Of the 2422 women, 844 had twin gestations, with 280 in the weekly contact group, 277 in the daily contact group, and 287 in the daily contact with home uterine activity monitoring group.

All of the women were asked to assess themselves for symptoms and signs of preterm labor and to palpate themselves for uterine contractions for 1 hour twice daily. The uterine activity monitoring group transmitted their data twice daily for immediate evaluation. Women who reached or exceeded their contraction thresholds or had symptoms or signs of preterm labor were asked to lie down, keep themselves hydrated, and palpate (or monitor) for another hour. If the signs and symptoms persisted or the contractions continued to exceed their thresholds, the patients were told to call the preterm labor center for evaluation and further directions.

The results of the study revealed that there were no significant differences among the groups in the incidence of birth at less than 35 weeks' gestation. In addition there were no significant differences in the amount of cervical dilatation at the time preterm labor was diagnosed, nor were there any significant differences in such neonatal outcomes as birthweight of less than 1500 g or less than 2500 g. However, of interest was that more-intensive surveillance promoted more unscheduled visits to the provider's office and a greater prophylactic use of tocolytic drugs in women who had some symptoms of preterm labor and contractions but who did not meet the criteria for a diagnosis of preterm labor. The additional unscheduled visits and the use of tocolytic drugs did not improve clinical outcomes.

Findings	Weekly Contact ($n = 798$)	Daily Contact ($n = 796$)	Daily with UA Monitoring ($n = 828$)
Incidence of birth <35 weeks	14%	13%	14%
Cervical dilatation at diagnosis of preterm labor	1.8 cm	1.5 cm	1.4 cm
Number of unscheduled visits	1.2	1.8	2.3
Prescribed tocolytic drugs	12%	14%	19%

In this study, for both the at-risk singleton and twin pregnancies, neither the addition of daily contacts with a nurse nor home monitoring of uterine activity provided additional benefits in terms of preventing preterm delivery, compared with education, daily uterine self-palpation, and weekly contact with a nurse among the culturally diverse, well-educated, and predominantly middle-class women who were participants in the study. In addition, daily contact and home monitoring increased the number of unscheduled visits and the prophylactic administration of tocolytic drugs without improving outcomes.

Other studies (Brown, 1999; CHUMS, 1995; Dyson et al, 1991; Iams, Johnson, O'Shaugnessy, 1988; Porto et al, 1987) have found that there was no difference in the detection of preterm labor with the use of a home monitoring device, contrasted with frequent contact with a nurse for 5 to 7 days each week. The results of the Dyson et al (1998) study are consistent with those findings, with the addition of not finding any significant differences between daily and weekly telephone contact with the patient. The use of home uterine activity monitoring and the frequency of contact with a nurse, as well as increases in unscheduled visits and prescription of prophylactic tocolytic drugs, should be considered in terms of competition for limited monetary resources. Further studies may provide additional information as the health care community seeks to reduce the number of preterm births, which are a major cause of perinatal morbidity and mortality.

Care of the Monitored Patient

9

Use of electronic fetal monitoring for antepartum and intrapartum patients is a standard of care for both low- and high-risk pregnancies. Also considered the standard of care is the use of electronic fetal monitoring in high-risk pregnancies for Non-Stress Testing (NST) and stress testing during the antepartum period. It is an expectation that nurses maintain adequate tracings and interpret baseline characteristics and periodic and nonperiodic changes. It is a standard of care for nurses to identify various patterns; document assessments, interpretations, and interventions; and notify appropriate people (e.g., obstetricians, neonatologists, and midwives) in a timely manner. Failure to do otherwise is practicing below the standard of practice and leaves nurses liable for their action or inaction.

One must keep in mind that the electronic fetal monitor, regardless of its level of sophistication, is only one tool used for fetal surveillance. A fetal heart rate (FHR) tracing should never be the only assessment method used to determine fetal well-being. Other assessment data that must be interpreted concurrently with the tracing include subjective data obtained from the patient and/or family during the admission interview, objective findings acquired from physical examination of the patient, laboratory data, results of any ultrasound examinations, and other pertinent data obtained from the patient's prenatal record.

The care given to the continuously monitored patient in labor is the same care given to any patient during labor, with additional consideration to those factors that relate directly to the monitor. The most important item by far is a thorough explanation to the patient and her partner and support people about the monitor—how it is used, how it is applied, and what is being evaluated.

Many patients are anxious about the status of the baby, concluding that something must be wrong that necessitates the monitor use. Some patients fear the machine itself and are distracted by its mechanical noises and beeps. Others are afraid to move in bed for fear of dislodging the leads and are concerned that the leads may harm the baby.

The health care provider must focus on the way in which people of different cultures and ethnicities perceive life events, the health care system, and the birthing process. To be effective, patient care must be provided in a culturally sensitive manner.

The digital display of FHR is also frequently a source of anxiety. Because the electronic fetal monitor cannot print out every heartbeat, sampling of FHR is displayed and often very low or very high numbers are observed. Patients expressing concern over these numbers should be told that variations in the displayed FHR are to be expected.

Often, the monitor is reassuring to the patient. An audible "beep" of the fetal heart sounds can be reassuring that all is well with the fetus. This sound often serves as encouragement to the patient, especially during active labor, when some patients, overwhelmed by their discomfort, lose sight of the imminent birth of their baby. For those patients who feel discouraged about labor, it is often reassuring to see evidence of uterine contractions. Visualizing contractions can also help the support person guide the laboring patient through the contraction by using breathing, focus, and relaxation techniques.

There is no contraindication to showing the patient and her support person the monitor strip differentiating FHR from uterine activity. Even when this is not shown to them, they quickly identify and contrast the FHR from the uterine activity (UA) panel without much difficulty. Patients do observe changes in the monitoring pattern, such as those caused by fetal movement, and can be given appropriate explanations when decelerations or dips in the FHR occur. After all, in an emergency there are no real secrets about the urgency of the situation.

Whether a patient is continuously monitored during labor or monitored for periods during labor, the care and issues involving documentation are the same. The monitor should not receive more attention than the patient (Figure 9-1). During the antepartum and intrapartum periods, the obstetrical nurse is responsible for two patients, maternal and fetal. This necessitates the use of both mater-

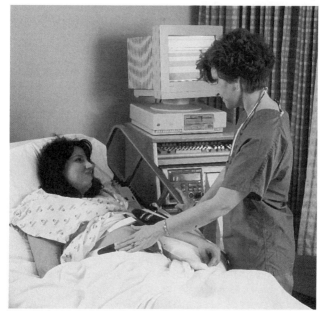

Figure 9-1
The nurse manages the care of the monitored patient,
ensuring that the monitor does not receive more attention
than the patient.
(Courtesy GE Marquette Medical Systems, Milwaukee, Wis.)

nal and fetal surveillance, which includes risk assessments determined through history taking, physical examination, and biochemical and biophysical testing. Laboring patients are monitored
for progress of labor, maternal well-being, pain management, psychosocial evaluation, and cultural needs. Intrapartum surveillance
evaluates fetal tolerance of labor and determines fetal well-being.
Guidelines for care are described in the following quick-reference
outline.

Care of the Monitored Patient

(See Appendix E for guidelines of basic patient care during the intrapartum period.)

Preparation of the Electronic Fetal Monitor

■ Test monitor as described by manufacturer and defined by hospital policy. Review Table 9-1 for an example of an equipment checklist.

■ Verify fetal monitor date/time with room clock or computer clock if using electronic documentation. The electronic fetal monitor clock should have the same time as whatever clock you are using in your documentation, such as time of birth.

■ Check transducers to ensure cleanliness and good working order.

Admission, Assessment, and Evaluation Process

■ Review of prenatal records, including laboratory and ultrasound data.

■ Vital signs, including temperature, respiration, pulse, and blood pressure.

■ Vaginal examinations, including cervical effacement, dilatation and station, and fetal presentation and position.

■ Status of membranes. If rupture of membranes has occurred before admission, document date/time of rupture of membrane, amount, odor if any, and color of fluid.

■ Patient views on pain management.

■ Uterine activity, including contraction onset, frequency, duration, and intensity.

■ Fetal heart baseline rate, variability, presence or absence of periodic or nonperiodic changes.

■ Provide information to the patient and her family about the electronic fetal monitor. This may include reason for monitoring, where the transducers will be located on the abdomen, and what information can be obtained from them.

■ An explanation of central monitoring and/or bedside electronic documentation.

■ Other assessments/observations may be included in the admission assessment as the patient's condition warrants.

Ongoing Care

Position patient comfortably

Encourage lateral position if bed is flat (modify this if patient is in semi-Fowler's position) to prevent supine hypotension syndrome

Assess progress of labor

Table 9-1   Fetal monitoring equipment checklist

Name: _____	Evaluator: _____		
Date: _____			

Items To Be Checked	Yes	No	Remarks
Preparation of Monitor 1. Is the paper inserted correctly? 2. Are the transducer cables plugged securely into the appropriate port?			
Ultrasound (US) Transducer 1. Has US transmission gel been applied to the transducer? 2. Was the FHR tested and noted on the monitor strip? 3. Does a signal light flash or an audible beep sound with each heartbeat? 4. Is the belt secure and snug but comfortable?			
Tocotransducer 1. Is the tocotransducer firmly positioned where there is the least maternal tissue? 2. Has the tocotransducer been applied without gel or paste? 3. Was the UA button/knob adjusted between the 10- and 20-mm marks and noted on the monitor paper? 4. Was this setting done between contractions? 5. Is the belt secure and snug?			
Spiral Electrode 1. Are the wires attached firmly to the leg plate? 2. Is the spiral electrode attached to the presenting part of the fetus? 3. Is the inner surface of the leg plate covered with electrode paste (if necessary)? 4. Is the leg plate properly secured to the patient's thigh?			

Continued

Table 9-1   Fetal monitoring equipment checklist—cont'd

Name: _____   Evaluator: _____
Date: _____

Items To Be Checked	Yes	No	Remarks
Intrauterine Pressure Catheter (IUPC)			
1. Is the length line on the catheter visible at the introitus?			
2. Is it noted on the monitor paper that a test or calibration was done?			
3. Has the monitor been set to zero according to the manufacturer's directions?			
4. Is the IUPC properly secured to the patient?			
5. Is baseline resting tone of uterus documented?			

Provide comfort measures/pain management per patient's preference

Record all nursing and patient care activities on monitor strip

During the active stage of labor

Document FHR q30min (in low-risk patients)

When risk factors are present, document FHR q15min when intermittent auscultation is used; if the patient is electronically monitored, the monitor strip should be evaluated q15min and initialed to verify this

During the second stage of labor

In low-risk patients the FHR should be documented q15min (if auscultated) or the monitor strip reviewed, evaluated, and initialed for patients who are electronically monitored

Evaluate and record the FHR q5min when auscultation is used in patients with risk factors

Evaluate the FHR monitor strip on electronically monitored patients with risk factors q5min

Document FHR immediately after membranes rupture and again in 5 minutes

External Monitoring
Ultrasound (US) Transducer

(Monitors FHR with high-frequency sound waves)

Use *Leopold's maneuvers* to assist in determining fetal lie to clearly locate FHR

Tap transducer gently with finger before use to ensure sound transmission

Apply ultrasound transmission gel to maternal abdomen

Clean abdomen and transducer and reapply gel prn

Massage reddened skin areas and reposition belt prn

Auscultate FHR with Doppler or fetoscope if in doubt as to the validity of monitor strip and compare with maternal pulse

Position and reposition transducer as needed to ensure clear, interpretable FHR data; massage reddened areas prn

Tocotransducer

(Monitors uterine activity via a pressure-sensing device placed on the maternal abdomen) (Figure 9-2)

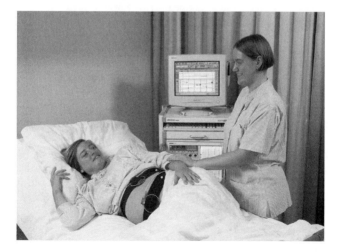

Figure 9-2
Externally monitored patient in lateral position.
(Courtesy Agilent Technologies, Böblingen, Germany.)

Palpate abdomen and position and reposition tocotransducer as needed on the fundus where the least maternal tissue is in evidence

Maintain snug abdominal belt

Adjust UA button/knob *between* contractions to print between 10 and 20 mm Hg on the monitor strip

Palpate fundus every 30 to 60 minutes to gauge strength of contraction; frequency and duration of contractions can be assessed only with tocotransducer

Do not assess patient's need for analgesia based on uterine activity displayed on strip; listen to patient's subjective viewpoint regarding contraction intensity, resting tone, and level of pain

Reposition belt and transducer and massage reddened skin areas prn; document and avoid areas of skin breakdown

Internal Monitoring

Spiral Electrode

(Obtains fetal ECG from presenting part and converts to FHR)

Connect spiral electrode to leg plate/cable per manufacturer's directions (e.g., one wire versus two wires, use of ECG paste versus ECG patch, use of leg belt versus a Velcro strap).

Apply electrode paste to leg plate prn, unless ECG patch is used

Observe FHR panel of monitor strip for variability

Turn electrode counterclockwise to remove; *never* pull straight out from presenting part

Administer perineal care as indicated

Intrauterine Pressure Catheter (IUPC)

(Catheter internally monitors intrauterine pressure)

Ensure that length line on catheter is visible at introitus

Zero the monitor according to the manufacturer's instructions

For fluid-filled catheters, release pressure valve of strain gauge, flush IUPC, and set uterine activity baseline to 0 line on monitor paper; test further as needed, according to manufacturer's instructions

Check proper functioning by tapping catheter, asking patient to cough, or applying fundal pressure; observe appropriate inflection on monitor strip

Keep catheter or cable secured to patient's leg to prevent dislodgment

Patient Teaching

Ensure that the patient and her support person(s) know and understand that the:

Use of the monitor does not imply fetal jeopardy

Fetal status via FHR can be continuously assessed even during contractions

Lower panel on the strip chart shows uterine activity and upper panel shows FHR

The volume on the FHR monitor can be turned up or down per patient's preference

The FHR sound and/or tracing may not be audible nor visible for short periods because of fetal or maternal movement

When using the external tocotransducer, the numbers on the uterine activity panel do not reflect the actual intensity of the contraction

The paper speed on the monitor is a reflection of time (e.g., 3 cm/min speed is 3 minutes of time; 1 cm/min speed is 1 minute of time; show where the vertical lines reflect the time frame)

If there is a bedside electronic documentation/central surveillance system, explain how you will be using it; show the patient which display is her fetal monitor tracing and how her labor can be monitored by staff when no one is physically present in the room

Prepared childbirth techniques can be implemented without difficulty

Effleurage performed during external monitoring can be done on the sides of the abdomen or upper thighs

Breathing patterns based on timing and intensity of contraction can be enhanced by observation of the uterine activity panel of the strip chart for onset of contractions

Note peak of contraction; knowing that contraction will not get stronger and is half over is usually helpful

Note diminishing intensity

Coordinate with appropriate breathing and relaxation techniques

Use of internal mode of monitoring does not restrict patient movement

Use of external mode of monitoring usually requires patient cooperation in positioning and movement

Documentation

Frequency of Fetal Heart Rate Evaluation

The frequency of documenting and evaluating the fetal heart rate during labor is based on standards of practice and on the risk assessment of the patient at the time of admission. The following frequencies are based on guidelines from the American Academy of Pediatrics and American College of Obstetricians and Gynecologists (1997). These frequencies are also recommended by the American Association of Women's Health, Obstetric and Neonatal Nurses (1997).

Stage of Labor	Low Risk	High Risk
Latent phase	q 30-60 minutes	q 30 minutes
Active phase	q 30 minutes	q 15 minutes
Second stage	q 15 minutes	q 5 minutes

Patient Care Documentation

The adage "if it was not documented, then it was not done" clearly applies to fetal monitoring and care of the patient in labor, especially when this information may be reviewed months or years later in legal action. It is imperative to have excellent records (Figure 9-3). Information that should be included follows:

1. Initiation of monitoring
   a. Patient's name and age
   b. Medical record number
   c. Date
   d. Midwife's or physician's name
   e. Time the monitor was attached and mode
   f. Testing/calibration
   g. Gravida _____ Para _____
   h. Expected date of confinement (EDC)
   i. Risk factors (e.g., pregnancy-induced hypertension, diabetes)
   j. Membranes intact or ruptured
   k. Gestational age
   l. Dilatation and station
2. During the course of monitoring
   a. Maternal position and repositioning in bed
   b. Vaginal examination and results

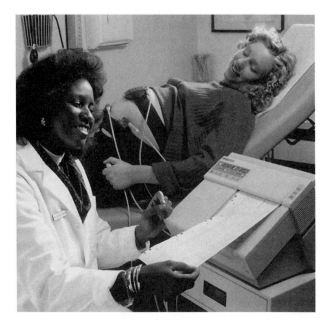

Figure 9-3
Documentation is easily achieved by hand-writing notes
directly on the tracing in this slant-top monitor.
(Courtesy Agilent Technologies, Böblingen, Germany.)

    c. Analgesia or anesthesia
    d. Medication/parenteral fluids
    e. Blood pressure, temperature, pulse, and respirations
    f. Voidings
    g. Oxygen given
    h. Emesis
    i. Pushing
    j. Fetal movement
    k. Any change in mode of monitoring
    l. Adjustments of equipment
        (1) Relocation of transducers
        (2) Type and adjustment of catheter
        (3) Replacement of electrode
        (4) Replacement or removal of IUPC/IUPT
        (5) Flushing of IUPC/IUPT

    m. Identification of nonreassuring FHR patterns
       If you know what it is—name it
       If the pattern is unknown—describe it
       If the pattern is indescribable—draw it
    n. Interventions for nonreassuring FHR patterns
      (1) Amnioinfusion
      (2) $FSpO_2$ monitoring
      (3) Scalp pH
      (4) Repositioning
      (5) O_2 administration
      (6) Medications administered or discontinued

The time of all aspects of care should be noted if the monitor does not automatically print the time. Initialling the monitor strip at designated intervals ensures that someone has assessed the patient and FHR on a regular basis and that any identified nonreassuring pattern has been identified and managed. The clarity and accuracy of documentation is important for performance improvement and teaching purposes and is of the utmost importance in identifying the cause of a specific FHR response to interventions.

3. On completion of monitoring and delivery, the nurse should make the following summary notations:
    a. Delivery date and time
    b. Type of delivery
    c. Anesthesia
    d. Gender and weight of the infant
    e. Presentation
    f. Both 1- and 5-minute Apgar scores
    g. Maternal or neonatal complications
    h. Presence or absence of meconium, character of meconium if present
    i. Cord blood pH, if done

This documentation contributes to a complete picture of the patient's labor.

Documentation during the intrapartum and postpartum period should include all routine aspects of assessment, diagnoses, interventions, and evaluation of patient care based on current standards of practice. Preprinted medical record forms for the perinatal patient are available from different companies, such as the Maternal/Newborn Record System (Hollister, Libertyville, Ill.), and professional organizations, such as The American College of

Obstetricians and Gynecologists (Washington, D.C.). In order to promote efficiency and consistency in documentation, a table or checklist format is used, which, although time-saving, more importantly provides a comprehensive overview of the patient.

Computer-based documentation systems are available as well and provide archival and retrieval capabilities. They are usually available from the companies that manufacture fetal monitors, as well as other companies such as the WatchChild system (Hill-Rom, Batesville Ind.) (Figure 9-4). With the advent of computer-based documentation systems, the process of documenting patient care across the perinatal continuum has become streamlined and efficient. Multiple data entry points in the outpatient and inpatient setting, the combination of concurrent fetal surveillance and documentation, system interfaces with fetal and maternal monitors, and the ability to obtain statistical reports optimize the time and effectiveness of the perinatal nurse/midwife and physician and the managers who support the clinical service. Statistical information can be used to perform outcome studies and identify and monitor areas

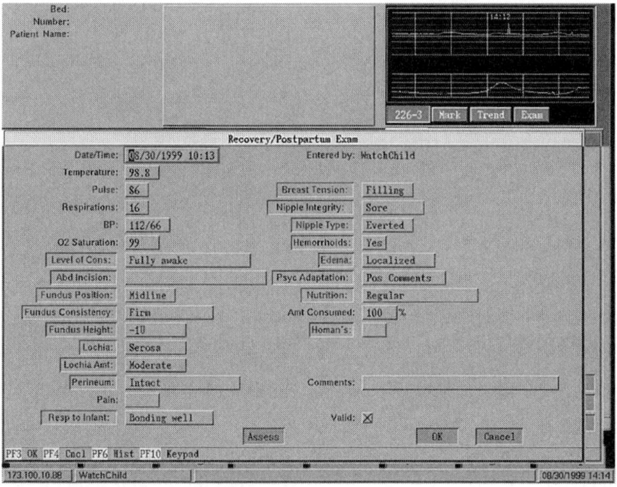

Figure 9-4

Monitor screen showing nursing documentation of routine assessment and postpartum care.

(Courtesy WatchChild, Hill-Rom Co. Inc., Batesville, Ind.)

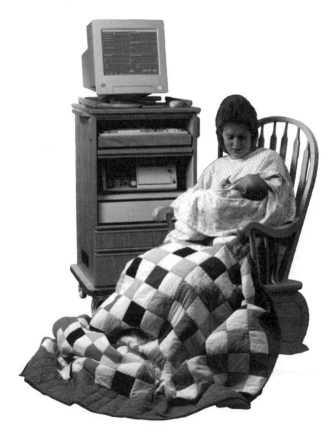

Figure 9-5
The desired outcome of quality patient care: a healthy postpartum patient and newborn.
(Courtesy WatchChild, Hill-Rom Co. Inc., Batesville, Ind.)

for improvement. In addition, this information can be used to meet the requirements of the state or province regulators and accrediting bodies. The benefits of a clear and complete record of the patient's care cannot be undervalued (Figure 9-5). Documentation systems, both paper-based and computer-based are discussed from a risk management perspective in Chapter 10.

Risk Management 10

Competency

The nurse/midwife is legally responsible for performing fetal monitoring according to the established standard of care as defined by the employer and the nurse's professional education, medical practice, and professional organizations and the local state nurse practice act. Observations, evaluation, and intervention for the patient's symptoms, progress, and reactions are the nurse's responsibility within legally sanctioned confines. The nurse/midwife who develops expertise in monitoring and pattern recognition is held responsible for this expertise.

Increasing concern for competency in fetal monitoring has resulted in a trend toward the need for validating that competency, such as by a written certification examination. Electronic fetal monitoring is but one method of fetal assessment and is conceptually and practically a part of other clinical assessment techniques used to manage normal, high-risk, physiological, and pathophysiological processes that may occur during the antepartum and intrapartum periods.

Electronic fetal monitoring is one part of a group of competencies based on a continuum of knowledge that the nurse must possess to care for antepartum and intrapartum patients. With the intent of promoting competency in clinical nursing practice, the Association of Women's Health, Obstetric, and Neonatal Nurses (AWHONN) has developed a *Clinical Competencies and Education Guide: Antepartum and Intrapartum Fetal Heart Rate Monitoring* (1998). (See Appendix G.) The guidelines describe the core content of educational programs and clinical practicums for FHR monitoring. The guide is designed to support the achievement of competency in electronic fetal monitoring and is an excellent resource for the practicing nurse, nurse manager, or administrator, as well as the nursing educator (see Appendix G).

These AWHONN guidelines offer a way to categorize nursing responsibilities in electronic fetal monitoring. From closed claim and expert review, it is apparent that nursing responsibility, and therefore liability, seems to fall into the following categories: obtaining the data, interpretation of the data, nursing intervention based on the data, notification of the appropriate practitioner, and documentation.

Obtaining the Data

Whether electronic fetal monitoring is required for a particular patient is a clinical decision that is made prospectively using data available to the practitioner at the time of the decision. This decision is also based on the policies, procedures, and standards of practice in a given institution. Although the "standard of care" may not require the use of an electronic fetal monitor, it is incumbent upon the nurse to use it properly once it is placed into use.

Hours of an uninterpretable monitor tracing does not show that any standard of care has been met simply because an electronic fetal monitor was on the patient. The charge to the perinatal nurse is to obtain and maintain an adequate tracing of the fetal heart and uterine contractions. The nurse must also be able to identify technically inadequate tracings and take appropriate corrective action. If the nurse is unable to continuously monitor the fetal heart, the nurse should document the attempts to adjust the monitor and note the FHR per auscultation until an interpretable tracing can be obtained. If all efforts prove unsuccessful, the nurse should notify the patient's primary care provider so that alternative methods of assessing the FHR may be explored.

Care must also be taken to obtain an adequate uterine contraction tracing. In one claim that resulted in a $2.2 million settlement, only the Doppler transducer was applied, with no tocotransducer used for uterine contraction monitoring. The fact that the nurses failed to use the tocotransducer resulted in an inability to evaluate the nature of decelerations that became evident on the monitor strip. A prudent nurse would have taken steps to obtain a complete strip in order to appropriately evaluate fetal well-being.

Before the widespread use of Labor/Delivery/Recovery rooms (LDRs) there was a spate of cases in which electronic fetal monitoring had been discontinued too soon. These involved patients who had been electronically monitored throughout their labors, but upon being transferred to the traditional "delivery room" had their electronic monitor discontinued and not transported with the patient to the delivery room for continued monitoring. The AAP/ACOG guidelines are quite clear that the standard of practice for monitoring low-risk patients in the second stage of labor is to evaluate—by either auscultation or electronic fetal monitor—and record the FHR at least every 15 minutes. When risk factors are present, the FHR should be evaluated and recorded at least every 5 minutes when auscultation is used and should be evaluated at least every 5 minutes when electronic fetal monitoring is used. If the patient has been in labor and is to undergo a cesarean delivery, fetal surveillance should continue until the abdominal sterile preparation is begun. If internal FHR monitoring is in use, it should be continued until the abdominal sterile preparation is complete (AAP/ACOG, 1997). It is recommended that facilities develop a policy to cover such situations. The tendency to not apply the same standards of monitoring and documentation when the patient is transferred from the labor room to the delivery room must be avoided, because considerable time may elapse between the time that the patient is taken to the delivery room and the delivery itself (Harvey, Chez, 1997). The absence of any documentation whatsoever of FHR monitoring, either by auscultation or electronic means, makes a case very difficult, if not impossible, to defend against charges of nursing negligence.

Interpretation of Data

In a landmark 1981 California case a verdict was returned in favor of a 3½-year-old child who was severely brain damaged since birth. The hospital was found totally liable, and the physician was exonerated. The physician attached the fetal monitor and went into his office because everything on the monitor strip appeared to be normal. Within a short period, however, there appeared profound and persistent late decelerations. The nurse who was assigned to care for the patient had no education or training in electronic fetal monitoring and failed to interpret the presence of fetal distress on the monitor. The fetal monitor continued to display marked heart rate abnormalities up to the time that the nurse called the physician to come and deliver the baby when the patient was fully dilated. Although the physician delivered the baby as expeditiously as possible, the baby was severely depressed at birth and suffered profound brain damage. The nurse's deposition was particularly effective in proving that the nurse knew next to nothing about fetal monitor interpretation. Experts testified that a nurse working in Labor and Delivery should be able to interpret the information provided by a fetal monitor. The jury determined that the hospital had both indirect and direct liability in this case. The hospital was vicariously, or indirectly, liable for the nurse's failure to interpret the monitor strip accurately and directly liable for placing an incompetent nurse in Labor and Delivery (Rubsamen, 1993).

The AWHONN core competencies state that the nurse should be able to "identify baseline fetal heart rate and rhythm, variability, and the presence of periodic and nonperiodic changes," as well as be able to "interpret the findings and implement nursing interventions" (AWHONN, 1998). It is also established law that nurses owe a duty to the patient to possess skills appropriate to their nursing function and that they must use **reasonable** care in the exercise of those skills. These statements should make it clear that the nurse should be able to interpret fetal monitor tracings and treat nonreassuring FHR patterns with appropriate nursing intervention. As Dr. Barry Schifrin stated so succinctly: "To utilize the fetal monitor without the capacity to interpret the tracing is negligent" (Schifrin, Weissman, Wiley, 1985).

Nursing Intervention Based on the Data

Again, the AWHONN competencies state that the nurse will "interpret the findings and implement nursing interventions." Such interventions include the accepted nursing interventions of position change(s); oxygen administration; discontinuation of oxytocin; possible vaginal examination; and, often, the obtaining of further data.

Documentation of nursing intervention should include the time and type of interventions instituted, **what the patient(s) response was to the intervention,** and each time that the physician or primary caregiver was notified. Documentation of the patient response to the intervention is crucial in the medical record, both for documenting either resolution or a continuation of the findings and for substantiating the rationale for the plan of action.

A problem of nursing intervention—or lack of intervention—often seen on claim and expert review is that all of the above nursing interventions were instituted except that of the discontinuation of oxytocin. Such a finding in the face of a nonreassuring FHR pattern is almost always indefensible. If there is frank or suspected fetal distress, the oxytocin **must be discontinued** until there is some resolution of the problem. Virtually all nursing policies state that oxytocin should be discontinued in the face of hyperstimulation or a nonreassuring FHR pattern. Such policies usually spell out clearly that the above nursing interventions are to be instituted at the nurse's discretion based on predetermined protocols. Nurses are cautioned to know what their institution's policies are, to adhere to them, and to review and update such policies on a regular basis for appropriateness, clarity, consistency, and feasibility.

Notification of the Appropriate Practitioner

After identification of a nonreassuring pattern, the nurse's responsibility does not cease with nursing intervention alone. After the nurse has identified a nonreassuring pattern and instituted and documented appropriate nursing interventions, he or she is then responsible for notifying the physician or certified nurse-midwife. Once the physician or other practitioner has been notified of a nonreassuring pattern, the nurse can expect that person to respond. An institutional policy should be established for the nurse to follow should the physician/practitioner be unable to respond in a timely fashion. Should the physician be unfamiliar with monitoring or have differences in interpretation, the nurse must follow hospital protocol for resolving the conflict.

Because electronic FHR monitoring is a complex clinical process that requires a great deal of skill and training and involves individual interpretation, the potential for conflict exists in terms of professional judgement and decision making. Freeman, Garite, and Nageotte (1991) best describe it as ". . . a modality that is difficult to learn, difficult to interpret. It has become a major factor in malpractice litigation, where its inexact nature confuses attorneys and lay juries." Given fetal monitoring's imprecision and that interpretations can differ, a hospital policy that addresses conflict resolution and allows the nurse to activate the facility's chain of command is an absolute necessity so that the patient receives timely medical attention (McRae, 1993).

A common scenario often put forth is that of the nurse who reports nonreassuring FHR patterns from observed findings on a FHR tracing. The physician, not at the bedside, disputes the nurse's interpretation. What subsequent steps should the nurse take?

It is important to remember that when a physician and nurse disagree, both have an obligation to the patient(s) to discuss and resolve the issue. In the "real world" of the clinical setting, this must be done quickly to facilitate appropriate treatment. The most appropriate way to resolve differences of opinion is usually contained in the facility's "chain of command or consultation" policy (Figure 10-1). Regardless, the staff nurse is often in a better position to speak with the physician about the matter if the nurse has reviewed the concerns with the charge nurse or another nurse recognized as a knowledgeable source. Such conversations should be documented, because they constitute a "nursing consultation" and can be very valuable from a defense point. Nurses do consultations all the time but rarely document them, unlike their medical colleagues who carefully record all consultations.

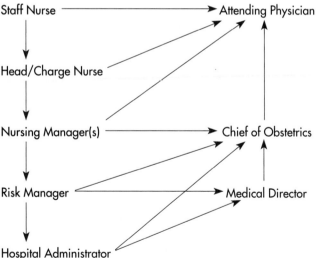

Figure 10-1
Sample chain-of-command/consultation for resolution of conflicts in judgment between nurse(s) and attending physician.

If, after discussion of the issue, the physician and nurse cannot resolve their differences and the nurse feels that she cannot carry out the resulting order, the dilemma should be presented to the charge nurse or supervisor. Generally, the next step is that the supervisor takes the issue to the chief of obstetrics. If the issue is unresolved, the risk manager should be notified. This lengthy "chain of command or consultation" approach is appropriate only when there is sufficient time available. An accelerated approach must be instituted if there is an emergent situation. The nurse must not waste time on the more passive-aggressive approach of "assumptions," as in "I assumed the physician was coming"; "I assumed the physician knew the need to be there right away"; and the ever-puzzling "I assumed the physician knew what I meant."

Nursing documentation should reflect that the physician was made aware of the FHR pattern and the time or times that the physician was notified.

Several years ago a California appellate decision, *Goff* v. *Doctors' Hospital* (1958), established the rule that a nurse has an independent professional duty to a patient. If it is within the nurse's professional competence to recognize that the doctor is neglecting the patient, and the patient may suffer because of it, that nurse has an obligation to use the chain of command to remedy the situation. The legal obligation of the nurse to utilize the facility's chain of command policy has been made very clear over the last few decades and has done much to do away with the antiquated legal theory of "Captain of the Ship."

Documentation and Retrieval

The importance of documentation on the patient's medical record cannot be overemphasized. Adherence to standards of practice is essential, and appropriate assessment, intervention, and evaluation should be clearly documented. The practitioner should anticipate how the patient's record may be analyzed by others years after a delivery, as occurs during the litigation process. The general assumption is that what is not written did not occur, and the concept of what the reasonable, prudent nurse would do in the same situation takes on a new meaning to those who become involved in medical or nursing malpractice.

The patient's medical record should include baseline information such as the time that the fetal monitor was applied and the mode of monitoring being utilized. Specific FHR information should include the baseline FHR, an estimation of baseline variability whenever possible, and the presence and type of periodic patterns.

Often overlooked, but equally important, are notations concerning baseline uterine resting tone and the presence, frequency, and duration of uterine contractions. Intensity of uterine contractions should be noted whenever an intrauterine pressure catheter is used.

It is appropriate to use the descriptive names that have been given to FHR patterns (e.g., accelerations and early, late, and variable decelerations) in written medical record documentation and verbal communication. The use of narrative description is indicated when the monitor tracing does not fit the established criteria for the usual descriptive names. Nurses are cautioned against the use of terms such as "fetal distress," "fetal hypoxia," or "uteroplacental insufficiency" in their charting because these terms are **medical** diagnoses, and there are no consensus definitions for these terms. ACOG's Committee on Obstetrical Practice (1995d) recommends replacing terms such as "fetal distress" with the term "nonreassuring fetal status," followed by further description of the findings.

If the findings on the monitor strip are nonreassuring, the nurse must embark on some course of remedial action and document those interventions and responses, as well as the time, or times, that the physician was notified of the pattern. Intervention notations should include the following:

- Time and type of nursing intervention initiated
- Patient response to the intervention
- The time(s) of physician notification and a summary of facts given to the physician. For example: "0535—Dr. Jones notified of the presence of late decelerations, which responded favorably to oxygen administration and position change"
- Any changes in the medical or nursing plan

Nurses should avoid the use of empty and meaningless charting phrases such as "physician notified of patient's condition." The chart should explain of what the physician was specifically notified. Such descriptive notes are invaluable should a problem arise years later. The following California case (Orimi, 1985) concerning perinatal brain damage illustrates this point all too clearly. The nurse had charted "Some decelerations noted; doctor advised of patient's condition." Questions arose during the discovery phase of litigation concerning the following: did the nurse telephone the obstetrician? (He did not recall speaking to her.) If she did call, what did she say? At the time of her deposition and testimony, she could not remember what she had or had not said to the obstetrician. The physician stated that had he only known of the decelerations, he would have gone immediately to the hospital to evaluate the patient. The jury accepted the physician's statement and the assertion by him that the nurse had provided too little information. The outcome of the trial was that the hospital was solely liable for damages totaling $5.8 million.

The overall goal of narrative medical record charting is to be accurate, objective, and free from editorial commentary, potentially damaging and biased comments, and "finger pointing." The medical record should never be used as the "battleground" but rather the means by which the health care professional can provide a clear, detailed, and objective account of the events as they occurred.

What goes in the patient's medical record and what goes on the strip chart? Do nurses have to record everything in both places? These questions arise from valid concerns about nurses having to chart the same or similar information on multiple chart forms. The goal should be to make charting time efficient without sacrificing accuracy and completeness. The fetal monitor strip can be viewed as a convenient bedside flow sheet on which to record all patient- or provider-initiated activities related to patient care. Examples of these activities include the following:

- Maternal status data, such as vital signs, activity or position changes, vaginal examination findings, or status of membranes
- Medications, including route, dosage, and time; medications may include analgesia or anesthesia, oxytocin, or tocolytics
- Nursing interventions, such as position changes, oxygen administration, discontinuation of oxytocin, vaginal examination findings, or hydration
- Delivery information, such as time and type of delivery, and baby information including sex, Apgar scores, weight, and any neonatal findings

When reviewing monitor strips, it is disturbing to see hours of monitor tracing with no entries whatsoever on the strip. Such a tracing may suggest that no one observed that patient for the entire time, which is, fortunately, rarely the case. Often, the nurse may have observed and even assessed the patient, then determined that no further nursing action was necessary at the time. Nurses should be encouraged to chart at least the time and their initials on the strip chart whenever they are at a patient's bedside. A policy should be established at each facility as to how often the tracing should be initialed when no scheduled patient care activities are taking place so as to document the physical presence or observation of the caregiver.

All FHR monitor strips should be labeled with identifying patient information. Several companies have developed standardized stick-on labels for this purpose. Subsequent labeling should take place when changing paper or switching monitors or when a health care provider tears off a piece of strip for any reason, because such actions result in a break in the continuous record. Each new segment should be labeled with the patient's name and the date and time. It is also helpful to note, on the beginning of a new paper pack, the number of the last paper panel. Sequential parts of the record should be labeled so that all pertinent information can be retained and reassembled. Whenever monitoring is initiated, at the change of shift, or at the beginning of a new paper pack, the nurse should make certain that the clock on the fetal monitor is in sync with the hospital clock. Many an hour has been spent by defense and plaintiff counsels and their experts trying to make sense of confusing discrepancies in times on FHR monitor strips and medical records.

Claims experience has shown that if the fetal monitor tracings or any portion of them are missing, the claim has become virtually indefensible. Each year hospitals or their liability insurance carriers pay hundreds of thousands of dollars in settlements for claims in which the case may have been otherwise entirely defensible. The issue is of one economics, as well as liability. The loss of fetal monitor strips may also expose the hospital to potential punitive damages because of allegations of fetal monitoring strips being purposefully destroyed (*Cedars-Sinai* v. *Superior Court,* 1996).

A properly documented monitor strip should be able to stand alone with the information contained on it. However, the medical record should also be able to stand alone, because monitor strips can and do disappear. The hospital medical records department is responsible for protecting hospital records from loss, defacement, tampering, and access by unauthorized individuals. FHR monitor strips are often critical to the defense of an obstetrical malpractice case and should be preserved in accordance with applicable statutes of limitation (ECRI, 1995). Ideally the monitor strips should be kept with the maternal medical record. Because of the bulkiness of electronic fetal monitor tracings, they are sometimes stored separately. If that is the case, they must be retrievable and care must be taken to ensure their integrity. For example, heat and humidity in some storage areas can eradicate tracings on heat-sensitive paper. Some fetal monitoring systems provide computerized documentation of the patient's FHR monitor strip in addition to the paper tracing provided at the patient's bedside (Figures 10-2, 10-3, and 10-4). Such systems allow entry of information onto the computerized tracing by light pen, keyboard, or bar-code scanner. In addition, storage on optical disks has met with satisfaction in

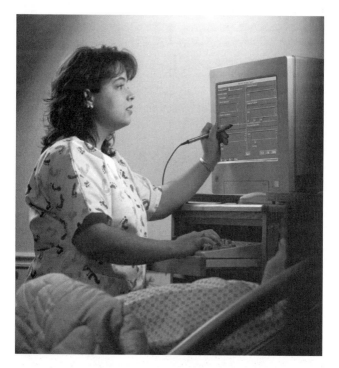

Figure 10-2
Nurse entering patient information into computer-based documentation system that interfaces with fetal/maternal monitors.
(Courtesy WatchChild, Hill-Rom Co. Inc., Batesville, Ind.)

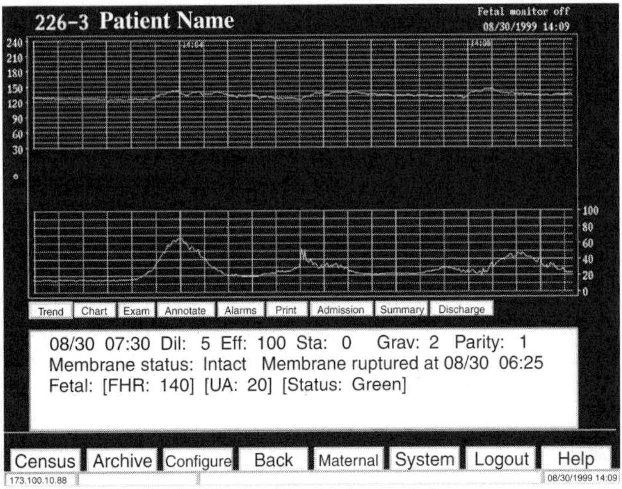

Figure 10-3
Monitor screen with documentation of patient's status in labor.
(Courtesy WatchChild, Hill-Rom Co. Inc., Batesville, Ind.)

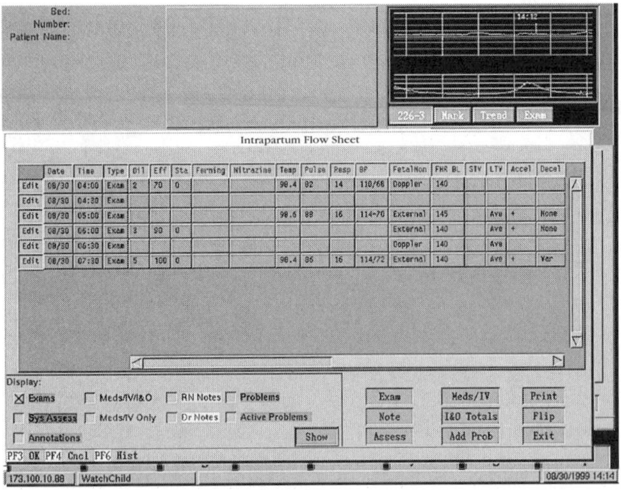

Figure 10-4
Monitor screen with flow sheet of patient's progress in labor.
(Courtesy WatchChild, Hill-Rom Co. Inc., Batesville, Ind.)

some facilities for storage, retention, and retrieval. Physicians, nurses, and administrators should be aware of their particular state's statutory regulations concerning the admissibility of computer-generated medical records in case of litigation. For facilities with limited storage space and without a computerized system, the use of microfilm may be preferred for improved retention of tracings and ease of storage.

As with any medical procedure, the patient has the right to refuse consent to be monitored. If a patient refuses the use of electronic fetal monitoring, the medical record should reflect that a thorough explanation of the reasons for its use and its benefits has taken place. The explanation of risks, benefits, and alternatives and the risks of refusing a given procedure are all part of the informed consent process, which remains the nondelegable duty of the physician. Therefore the nurse must be certain that the physician is notified if a patient refuses monitoring. The medical record must then note that the patient understands the explanation that she has been given. If new risk factors develop, the patient should be given an explanation of the new indications and the explanation should be documented again. The record must reflect that a truly informed consent—or refusal—has taken place. As the patient advocate, it is the duty of the nurse to ascertain whether that process has taken place and to notify the physician to remedy the situation if it has not.

The goal of fetal monitoring is to prevent or minimize potential fetal and maternal risk or injury. Adequate electronic fetal monitoring documentation facilitates assessment of maternal and fetal responses to nursing intervention, medication, and stresses such as uterine contractions. As with any documentation, it needs to be factual, objective, and timely. Careful documentation is essential to accurately reflect the quality of the care provided. Its importance has taken on greater significance because of the current malpractice environment.

Appendix A

High-Risk Factors

Antepartum maternal and fetal factors as well as intrapartum factors can increase maternal and fetal/neonatal risk. Early identification of these factors is needed to provide the direction for patient care management.

Medical History and Conditions

Anemia

Antiphospholipid syndrome

Asthma

Cancer

Cardiac disease

Collagen diseases (e.g., systemic lupus erythematosus [SLE], rheumatoid arthritis, scleroderma)

Condylomata, extensive

Diabetes mellitus, type 1 or 2

Domestic violence/intimate partner abuse

Drug addiction or alcohol abuse

Epilepsy

Family history of genetic disorders

Hemoglobinopathy

Human immunodeficiency virus (HIV)

Hypertension

Immunological disorders (autoimmune and alloimmune)

Neurological disorder

Nutritional status, poor

Psychiatric illness

Pulmonary disorders

Renal disease

Scoliosis

Smoking

Thromboembolic disease

Thyroid disease

Urinary tract infection
Uterine leiomyomata or malformation
Obstetric History and Conditions
Abnormal fetal presentation
Age >35 at delivery
Decreased fetal movement
Fetal cardiac malformation
Fetal growth restriction
Fetal anomalies (e.g., anencephaly)
Gestational age >41 weeks
Gestational diabetes
HELLP (hypertension, elevated liver enzymes, and low platelet counts) syndrome
Herpes, active lesions
Hydramnios
Incompetent cervix
Isoimmunization
Intrauterine growth restriction
Emotional instability
Lack of prenatal care
Low income
Marginal separation of placenta
Multiparity
Multiple gestation, especially with discordant growth
Nonimmune hydrops
Oligohydramnios
Preeclampsia
Pregnancy-related hypertension
Preterm labor
Premature rupture of membranes
Previous cesarean delivery
Prior fetal structural or genetic disorder
Prior unexplained fetal death
Prior neonatal death
Prior preterm delivery
Prior low birth weight (<2500 g)
Proteinuria
Sexually transmitted disease (STD), untreated
Systemic disease that has an adverse impact on pregnancy
Vaginal bleeding

Intrapartum Factors

Abnormal antenatal test
Abruptio placentae
Assisted vaginal delivery; vacuum or forceps
Amnionitis
Dysfunctional labor pattern
General anesthesia
Hemorrhage
Illicit drug use
Low birth weight, expected/actual
Maternal fever
Meconium in amniotic fluid
Nonreassuring fetal heart rate pattern
Oxytocin augmentation or induction of labor
Placenta previa
Precipitous labor
Preterm fetus
Postterm fetus
Prolapsed umbilical cord
Prolonged rupture of membranes >24 hours
Prolonged second stage of labor
Shoulder dystocia
Uterine hyperactivity/tetany
Uterine rupture

Appendix B

Leopold's Maneuvers and Determination of the Points of Maximal Intensity (PMI) of the Fetal Heart Rate

Leopold's Maneuvers

Wash hands.

Ask woman to empty bladder.

Position woman supine with one pillow under her head and with her knees slightly flexed.

Place small rolled towel under woman's right hip to displace uterus to left of major blood vessels (prevents supine hypotensive syndrome).

If right-handed, stand on woman's right, facing her:

1. Identify fetal part that occupies the fundus. The head feels round, firm, freely movable, and palpable by ballottement; the breech feels less regular and softer (identifies fetal lie [longitudinal or transverse] and presentation [cephalic or breech]; see figure below)

From Lowdermilk DL, Perry SE, Bobak IM et al: *Maternity nursing,* ed 5, St Louis, 1999, Mosby.

2. Using palmar surface of one hand, locate and palpate the smooth convex contour of the fetal back and the irregularities that identify the small parts (feet, hands, elbows). This assists in identifying fetal presentation (see figure below).

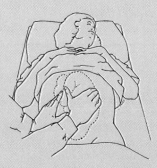

3. With the right hand, determine which fetal part is presenting over the inlet to the true pelvis. Gently grasp the lower pole of the uterus between the thumb and fingers, pressing in slightly (see figure below). If the head is presenting and not engaged, determine the attitude of the head (flexed or extended).

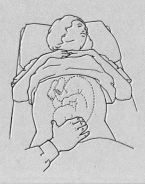

4. Turn to face the woman's feet. Using two hands, outline the fetal head (see figure below) with palmar surface of fingertips.

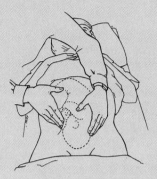

When presenting part has descended deeply, only a small portion of it may be outlined.

Palpation of cephalic prominence assists in identifying attitude of head.

If the cephalic prominence is found on the same side as the small parts, the head must be flexed, and the vertex is presenting. If the cephalic prominence is on the same side as the back, the presenting head is extended and the face is presenting.

Determination of PMI of FHR:

Wash hands.

Perform Leopold's maneuvers.

Auscultate FHR based on fetal presentation. The PMI is the location where the FHR is heard the loudest, usually over the fetal back.

Chart fetal presentation, position, and lie; whether presenting part is flexed or extended, engaged or free floating. Use hospital's protocol for charting (e.g., "Vtx, LOA, floating").

Chart PMI of FHR using a two-line figure to indicate the four quadrants of the maternal abdomen, right upper

quadrant (RUQ), left upper quadrant (LUQ), left lower
quadrant (LLQ), and right lower quadrant (RLQ):

RUQ	LUQ
RLQ	LLQ

The umbilicus is the point where the lines cross. The PMI
for the fetus in vertex presentation, in general flexion
with the back on the mother's right side, commonly is
found in the mother's right lower quadrant and is
recorded with an "x" or with the FHR as follows:

or

x	

140	

Appendix C

Protocols for the Initiation of Labor:
Cervical Ripening, Amniotomy, and
Oxytocin Augmentation/Induction

Cervical ripening is a complex process that culminates in the physical softening and distensibility of the cervix (ACOG, 1995b).

Amniotomy is the artificial rupture of the membranes.

Induction consists of stimulation of uterine contractions before the spontaneous onset of labor for the purpose of accomplishing delivery (ACOG, 1995b). Generally the induction of labor has merit as a therapeutic option when the benefits of expeditious delivery outweigh the risks of continuing the pregnancy (ACOG, 1999b).

Augmentation is the correcting of ineffective uterine contractions (caused by dystocia) that occur after the start of spontaneous labor (ACOG, 1995a).

Cervical Ripening

Cervical ripening changes the consistency of the uterus, making it softer and more distensible. This can be achieved by mechanical and chemical methods, including stripping of the membranes, use of hygroscopic dilators, and the application of prostaglandin E_2 gel. Cervical ripening is desirable whenever induction of labor is indicated, the cervix is not favorable for induction, and there are no contraindications to the use of cervical ripening agents.

Stripping of the Membranes

Stripping of the membranes involves the digital separation of the membranes from the lower uterine segment. This is achieved through a vaginal examination, often with simultaneous pressure on the fundus of the uterus to ensure application of the vertex on the cervix.

The effects of membrane stripping are inconsistent and more likely to be effective with a higher Bishop score.

Possible complications

Bleeding from low-implanted placenta
Infection
Rupture of membranes

Hygroscopic/Osmotic Dilators

Synthetic hygroscopic dilators and laminaria japonicum (seaweed stems) placed into the endocervix absorb fluid, expand, and cause a dilator effect on the cervix. A number of dilators can be inserted under direct visualization and are held in place with povidone-iodine saturated gauze sponges. Laminaria ripens the cervix but may be associated with increased peripartum infections (ACOG, 1999b).

Balloon Catheters

Balloon catheters have been used for cervical ripening for many years. A 24 French Foley catheter with a 30- to 50-ml balloon can be passed through an undilated cervix before inflation. Once in place the catheter is inflated with 30 ml of saline and then pulled back so that the bulb is hitched against the internal cervical os. The basic mechanism of cervical ripening by balloon seems to be direct pressure and overstretching of the lower uterine segment and cervix, and that overstretching results in increased prostaglandin concentrations in the amniotic fluid and maternal plasma. On release, the prostaglandins are involved in cervical softening and subsequent uterine contractions. The advantage of this method is its low cost and lack of need for fetal monitoring (Summers, 1997; Lurie, Rabinerson, 1997).

Prepidil (Dinoprostone)

Local application of prostaglandin E_2 gel (PGE_2) is a widely used cervical ripening agent. Prostaglandin E_2 gel placed onto the vagina or the cervical canal ripens the cervix, although intravaginal application may be more effective (Irion, Pedrazzoli, Mermillod, 1998). It should be administered only to patients for whom induction of labor is indicated.

Usual dosage

1. 0.5 mg when instilled in the endocervix
2. 2 to 3 mg when gel is placed intravaginally

Dinoprostone in a dosage of 0.5 mg is packaged in a prefilled syringe. A shielded catheter with a 10- or 20-mm tip is attached to the syringe to place the gel into the endocervix.

Guidelines for the use of dinoprostone gel

May be used up to 3 times, 6 to 12 hours apart within a 24-hour period

Should be applied by an appropriately credentialed health care provider

Caution should be exercised when using in patients with history of asthma; glaucoma; or pulmonary, hepatic, or renal disease

Use only in hospital setting when a physician who has delivery privileges to perform a cesarean delivery is readily available

Patient should be instructed to remain supine for 15 to 30 minutes to minimize leakage of gel

Store in refrigerator; warm to room temperature and prepare prostaglandin gel per supplier's instructions

Monitor patient for uterine hyperstimulation and FHR changes by palpation and auscultation or continuous electronic FHR monitoring for 2 hours

If hyperstimulation occurs, turn patient to lateral position, administer oxygen, and consider the use of a tocolytic agent

Hyperstimulation is defined as either a series of single contractions lasting 2 minutes or more, or a contraction frequency of five or more in 10 minutes.

If oxytocin is required, it should not be started for at least 6 hours following the last gel application

Contraindications to prostaglandin gel

Patients in whom oxytocin is generally contraindicated

Patients with previous cesarean section with a classical incision or major uterine surgery

Patients with hypersensitivity to prostaglandins or constituents of the gel

Cervidil

The newest formulation of prostaglandin contains dinoprostone in a controlled-release vaginal insert. It was approved for use as a cervical ripening agent by the Food and Drug Administration (FDA) in 1995. Cervidil is a thin, flat, rectangularly shaped polymeric chip containing 10 mg of dinoprostone. The chip is encased within a pouch of knitted polyester with a removal cord.

Guidelines for the use of Cervidil

The vaginal insert should be stored in the refrigerator before use

Patients receiving Cervidil should have continuous FHR and uterine activity monitoring (can be off the monitor to ambulate to the bathroom) until at least 15 minutes after it is removed

The Cervidil vaginal insert is placed transversely in the posterior fornix of the vagina immediately after removal from its foil package

The insertion of the vaginal insert does not require sterile conditions

The vaginal insert must not be used without its retrieval system (string attached)

A minimal amount of lubricant may be used to assist in insertion

Care should be taken not to permit excess contact or coating with the lubricant and thus prevent optimal swelling and release of dinoprostone from the vaginal insert

Cervidil should be removed 12 hours after insertion or when active labor ensues

Precautions

Cervidil must be removed:

At least 30 minutes before oxytocin administration is initiated

Before amniotomy

Any evidence of uterine hyperstimulation, sustained uterine contraction, fetal distress, or other fetal or maternal adverse reactions, should be a cause for removal of the insert

Cytotec (Misoprostol)

Misoprostol (Cytotec) is a synthetic prostaglandin E_1 analogue that has been indicated for peptic ulcer prevention in patients taking nonsteroidal antiinflammatory drugs. Misoprostol has become an intensely investigated topic for labor induction and cervical ripening (Adair et al, 1998). Various authors have reported on its excellent efficacy, minimal side effects, and cost-saving benefits ($0.36 for a single tablet) (Adair et al, 1998). Misoprostol is less expensive, more stable, and easier to store than dinoprostone preparations (ACOG, 1999a). Misoprostol has much the same mechanism of action, benefits, complications, indications, adverse reactions, and contraindications as other cervical/vaginal prostaglandin products (e.g., Prepidil and Cervidil). It has been found to be somewhat more effective than dinoprostone (Sanchez-Ramos et al, 1998).

Guidelines for the use of misoprostol (Cytotec)

The patient should be examined before the administration of misoprostol

The fetus should be in the vertex presentation

Listed are two possible protocols for the use of misoprostol for cervical ripening and induction of labor (Bornstein, Shuwager, 1999; Zieman et al, 1997; and Benett et al, 1998)

Observe for uterine hyperstimulation

Protocol for vaginal dosing

- *Obtain a reactive NST*
- *Insert 25 to 50 µg misoprostol in the posterior vaginal fornix; NOTE: misoprostol is supplied in 100-µg tablets*
- *Monitor maternal vital signs and FHR in accordance with hospital policy and ACOG guidelines*
- *Can repeat dose every 3 to 6 hours up to a total of 6 doses*
- *Pitocin can be started 4 hours after the last dose of misoprostol*
- *After 3 to 4 hours the patient can ambulate*
- *Observe for signs of FHR changes and uterine hyperstimulation*

Protocol for oral dosing

- *Obtain a reactive NST*
- *Give 100-µg misoprostol tablet orally*
- *Monitor maternal vital signs and FHR in accordance with hospital policy and ACOG guidelines*
- *The dose can be repeated every 4 hours for up to 6 doses*
- *Pitocin can be started 4 hours after the last dose of misoprostol*
- *After 3 to 4 hours the patient can ambulate*
- *Observe for signs of FHR changes and uterine hyperstimulation*

Low-Dose Oxytocin Infusion

Oxytocin is considered a poor ripening agent; however, low-dose oxytocin administration may ripen the cervix.

Dosage

Starting dose: 0.5 milliunits per minute

Increase dose: 1 milliunit per hour

Maximum dose: 4 milliunits per minute

Amniotomy

The artificial rupture of membranes can be an effective method of initiating uterine contractions and labor when the cervix is favorable. The fetal head should be well applied to the cervix and well engaged to reduce the risk of umbilical cord prolapse. The FHR should be monitored before and after the procedure; the color (clear or meconium stained) of the amniotic fluid should be documented, as well as the amount and odor of the fluid. Delivery achieved within 24 hours reduces the risk of chorioamnionitis. Therefore if spontaneous labor has not begun within 12 hours of rupture of membranes, the administration of oxytocin may be considered. The maternal temperature should be monitored per facility policy but no less frequently than every 4 hours after the rupture of membranes. Signs of infection should be documented and reported in an expeditious manner; signs include fetal tachycardia, maternal fever, chills, and malodorous vaginal drainage.

Oxytocin Infusion: Augmentation or Induction of Labor

Oxytocin infusion may be used either to begin the labor process or augment a labor that is progressing slowly because of inadequate uterine activity. Indications for induction include but are not limited to the following:

Maternal indications
1. Pregnancy-induced hypertension
2. Premature rupture of membranes
3. Chorioamnionitis

4. Maternal medical problems (e.g., diabetes mellitus, renal disease, and chronic obstructive pulmonary disease, chronic hypertension)
5. Preeclampsia, eclampsia

Logistic reasons such as distance from hospital or risk of rapid labor and psychosocial indications may be considerations for the induction of labor. If this is done, confirmation of term gestation or fetal lung maturity should be made by preestablished criteria (ACOG, 1999b).

Fetal indications
1. Macrosomia
2. Fetal demise
3. Fetal anomaly
4. Blood group sensitization
5. Nonreassuring fetal testing
6. Fetal hydrops
7. Intrauterine growth restriction
8. Postterm gestation

Contraindications to induction
Include but are not limited to the following:
1. Placenta or vasa previa
2. Transverse fetal lie
3. Prolapsed umbilical cord
4. Previous transfundal uterine surgery (e.g., classical uterine incision)
5. Active genital herpes infection

Some obstetric situations are not contraindications to induction of labor but do require special attention. These include but are not limited to the following:
1. One or more previous low-transverse cesarean delivery
2. Breech presentation
3. Maternal heart disease
4. Multifetal pregnancy
5. Polyhydramnios
6. Presenting part above the pelvic inlet
7. Severe hypertension
8. Abnormal FHR patterns not necessitating emergent delivery

Assessment

Observations/Findings

Dysfunctional labor pattern (Table C-1)
Absence of cephalopelvic disproportion
Bishop score ≥6 (Table C-2)

Laboratory/Diagnostic Studies

FHR-uterine activity monitoring
Ultrasound

Potential Complications

Nonreassuring FHR patterns
    Late decelerations
    Prolonged deceleration

Table C-1   Dysfunctional labor patterns

Labor Pattern	Nulligravida	Multipara
Protraction Disorders		
Dilation	<1.2 cm/hr	<1.5 cm/hr
Descent	<1.0 cm/hr	<2.0 cm/hr
Arrest Disorders		
Dilation	>2 hr	>2 hr
Descent	>1 hr	>1 hr

From American College of Obstetricians and Gynecologists: *Dystocia and the augmentation of labor,* tech bull 218, Washington DC, Dec 1995a, The College.

Table C-2   Bishop scoring system

	Score			
Area of Assessment	0	1	2	3
Station of presenting part	−3	−2	−1/0	+1/+2
Dilatation (cm)	0	1-2	3-4	>5
Effacement (%)	0-30	40-50	60-70	≥80
Consistency	Firm	Medium	Soft	—
Position of os	Posterior	Central	Anterior	—

Severe variable decelerations
Absence of variability
Bradycardia
Uterine hyperstimulation
  Contractions longer than 90 seconds
  Contractions occurring more frequently than q2min (tachysystole)
  Inadequate uterine relaxation: less than 30 seconds between contractions
  Intrauterine resting tone: above 25 mm Hg pressure between contractions
  Sustained tetanic uterine contraction
Meconium passage
Maternal hypertension
Water intoxication
  Rising blood pressure
  Edema of face and fingers and around the eyes
  Difficulty breathing
  Urinary output <30 to 50 ml/hr
Abruptio placentae: sudden, severe uterine pain
Rupture of vasa previa
Precipitate delivery
Hemorrhage
Shock
Uterine rupture
Amniotic fluid embolism

Medical Management

Oxytocin infusion (ACOG, 1999b)
Low-dose regimens
1. Oxytocin at 0.5 to 1.0 mU/min and incremental increases for desired results at 30- to 40-minute intervals in increments of 1 mU/min *or*
2. Oxytocin at 1 to 2 mU/min and incremental increases of 2 mU/min every 15 minutes
High-dose regimens
1. Oxytocin at 6 mU/min with incremental increases of 6 mU/min every 15 minutes, *or*
2. Oxytocin at 6 mU/min with incremental increases at 6, 3, or 1 mU/min every 20 to 40 minutes

For 6 mU/min regimen, reduce the incremental increase to 3 mU/min in the presence of hyperstimulation and reduce to 1 mU/min with *recurrent* hyperstimulation

Evaluate for normal progression of labor with 150 to 350 Montevideo Units of uterine activity

Monitor FHR and uterine activity continuously, preferably with the internal mode of monitoring

Analgesia

Administer

Tocolytic agents for excessive uterine activity that persists after oxytocin is discontinued, supportive treatment provided (lateral position and oxygen by mask), and fetal distress is present

Terbutaline 0.25 mg IV push or magnesium sulfate 4 g, 10% solution over 15 to 20 minutes IV

Nursing Diagnoses/Interventions/Evaluation

▼Risk for injury related to an exogenous source of oxytocin

See Care of Patient in First Stage of Labor (Appendix E)

Maintain complete bed rest

Ensure that physician is immediately available

Apply fetal monitoring; obtain baseline strip before starting IV oxytocin and before application of ripening agent

Place patient in comfortable position; lateral position is preferred

Always piggyback oxytocin solution into main IV line close to needle insertion site (10 U oxytocin in 1000 ml IV fluid = 10 mU/ml)

Administer oxytocin via a controlled-infusion device as ordered

Monitor dose in mU/min q15min and before each increase

Increase rate of oxytocic solution as ordered to produce contractions q2min to 3min of 30- to 60-seconds duration

Monitor patency of parenteral system

Check BP, P, and FHR q15min to 30min or as ordered

Observe contractions for frequency, duration, strength, and relaxation q5min for five times, then q15min to 30min and prn

Administer analgesics as ordered

Assist in breathing and relaxation techniques

Encourage frequent position change

Measure intake and output q2h

Prepare for delivery as indicated

Reinforce provider's explanation of reason for augmentation or induction of labor

Expected outcome/evaluation

Mother and fetus are not compromised as a result of oxytocin infusion

Patient Teaching

Reinforce provider's explanations

Discuss indications for procedure

Explain methodology of administration

Discuss expected effects of oxytocin induction/augmentation of labor

Explain differences between induction/augmentation and normal, spontaneous contractions

Ensure that patient and significant other verbalize understanding of procedure, indications for it, and expected effects

Appendix D

Protocol for Management of Preterm Labor

Preterm Labor

Preterm labor is labor that occurs before completion of the thirty-seventh week of gestation. It is characterized by uterine contractions associated with documented changes in cervical parameters (ACOG, 1995e; ACOG 1998b).

Contraindications to Tocolysis

Maternal
    Abruptio placentae, severe
    Chorioamnionitis
    Severe antepartum vaginal bleeding
    Pregnancy-induced hypertension
    Prolonged ruptured membranes
Fetal
    Fetal demise
    Fetal anomalies incompatible with life
    Severe fetal growth restriction
    Documented fetal maturity
    Fetal condition in which prolongation of pregnancy is detrimental to fetal life

General Assessment
Subjective and objective data

Gestational age and fetal status
Uterine contractions
    Every 10 minutes or less (6 to 8 uterine contractions per hour)
    Lasting 30 seconds or more, preferably documented by toco-transducer
Progressive cervical dilatation: ≥50% effacement or ≥2 cm dilatation
Complaints of back pain or pressure
Possible spontaneous rupture of membranes

Confirmation of indication

Gestational age of at least 20 weeks but less than 37 weeks*

Regular uterine contractions at frequent intervals preferably documented by tocotransducer

Documented cervical change or appreciable cervical dilation or effacement

Laboratory/diagnostic studies

Electronic fetal monitoring

Fetoscope/Doppler

Urinalysis (rule out urinary tract infection)

CBC

Cervical cultures, including group B streptococcus (GBS)

Amniocentesis to assess fetal lung maturity and presence of infection

Maternal and fetal baseline ECG

Electrolytes

Blood glucose

C-reactive protein (CRP)

Fetal fibronectin (Goldenberg et al, 1996; Morrison et al, 1996; Peaceman, 1997; and Moore, 1999)

Potential complications

Compromised infant at birth
  Prematurity
  Small-for-gestational-age infant
  Respiratory distress syndrome

Multidisciplinary Management

Bed rest may be indicated; semi-Fowler's position preferred

Continuous electronic fetal monitoring and uterine contraction monitoring for a minimum of 1 hour

Home uterine activity monitoring as indicated by condition, uterine activity, fetal gestational age, and maternal compliance with regimen (Shellhass, Iams, 1998; Dyson et al, 1998)

Laboratory tests as indicated

Monitor BP, TPR as indicated

IV fluids as indicated

Intake and output

*Based on institutional policy.

Ultrasound for evaluation of placenta, fetal/uterine anomalies, and gestational age confirmation

Glucocorticoids (recommended for all patients in preterm labor between 24 and 34 weeks' gestation)

Tocolysis as indicated (magnesium sulfate, nifedipine, terbutaline, indomethacin, or ritodrine hydrochloride)

Antibiotics as indicated

General Guidelines in the Use of Tocolytics

Limit tocolytic treatment to women with both cervical change and regular uterine contractions before 34 to 35 weeks' gestation

If the first agent fails to produce tocolysis, use a second standard agent

Exercise caution with the combination of therapies

Use minimum amount of IV tocolytics for the shortest period of time

If tocolysis fails, consider:

Placental abruption

Chorioamnionitis

Unsuspected uterine malformation

Use indomethacin and calcium blockers only in special circumstances

Respect maternal and fetal contraindications to tocolysis

Follow established protocols

Drug mixing

Amount of drug per milliliter of parenteral fluid

Administration precautions

Specific Tocolytic Agents
Magnesium Sulfate
Contraindications

Hypocalcemia

Myasthenia gravis

Renal failure

Assessment

Maternal effects

Flushing, sense of warmth

Nasal stuffiness/congestion

Headache
Dizziness
Respiratory depression
Hypotension
Hyporeflexia
Nystagmus
Tetany (rare)
Nausea, vomiting
Lethargy, fatigue
Pulmonary edema
Fetal/neonatal effects
  Decreased muscle tone
  Respiratory depression
  Lethargy, drowsiness
  Lower Apgar scores with prolonged maternal treatment

Administration

Maintain patent IV access
Administer 3 to 6 g IV in a 10% solution over 15 to 30 minutes for initial dose as ordered
Continue and monitor IV infusion titrated according to uterine response and side effects (i.e., 2 g/hr)

Related patient care

Watch for symptoms of toxicity; discontinue infusion, administer oxygen therapy, and notify physician if toxicity occurs
  Respiratory depression
  Hypotension
  Absence of deep tendon reflexes
  Keep antidote for magnesium sulfate toxicity (10% calcium gluconate) at bedside
Monitor and decrease dosage after 24 hours or when uterine contractions subside as ordered
Check vital signs and deep tendon reflexes (DTRs) q30min to 1h
Continue to monitor uterine activity
Monitor intake and output q1h; should be at least 30 ml urine per hour
Auscultate lungs q4h to 8h for presence of fluid
Monitor fetus with electronic fetal monitoring as ordered
Check FHR with vital signs if no electronic fetal monitoring is done

Monitor magnesium sulfate levels
Obtain baseline electrolytes and calcium levels by venipuncture

Nifedipine
Contraindications

Maternal liver disease

Assessment

Maternal effects
  Slight flushing
  Slight hypotension
  Headache
  Nausea
  Peripheral edema
  Periorbital edema
  Syncope
Fetal/Neonatal effects
  Not determined

Administration

Oral administration
  Administer 10 mg PO; repeat in 20 minutes if still contracting
    and once again after 20 minutes if necessary; then 10 to 20 mg
    q4 to 6h
NOTE: Sublingual administration has been discontinued because of
  potential hypotension (Creasy, Iams, 1999)

β_2 Adrenergic Agents (Terbutaline and Ritodrine)
Contraindications

Maternal cardiac rhythm disturbance or other cardiac disease
Poorly controlled diabetes, thyrotoxicosis, or hypertension

Assessment: terbutaline

Maternal effects
  Tachycardia, palpitations
  Hypotension
  Arrhythmias
  Hypokalemia
  Chest pain
  Pulmonary edema
  Tremors, agitation

Headache
Elevated blood glucose
Hyperlipidemia
Fetal/neonatal effects
Fetal distress
Tachycardia
Bradycardia if severe maternal hypotension
Neonatal hypotension
Neonatal hypoglycemia
Neonatal hypocalcemia
Neonatal irritability

Assessment: ritodrine

Maternal and fetal/neonatal effects (same as terbutaline)

Administration: terbutaline

Parenteral administration
Administer loading dose of 0.25 mg slowly
For continued therapy add 15 mg terbutaline to 250 ml of D_5W
or NS (this will deliver 60 μg/ml)
Give 5 μg/min and increase dose in 5-μg increments q10 min
until tocolysis is achieved or until 55 μg/min is reached
Oral therapy
Administer first dose before discontinuing parenteral therapy
Dosage 2.5 to 5.0 mg q4h PO until 36 weeks' gestation
Subcutaneous administration
Administer 0.25 mg SQ, and repeat same dose in 30 min if uter-
ine contractions persist
For continued therapy give 0.25 mg SQ every 4 hours for 24
hours and then switch to oral therapy or per physician order
If birth occurs quickly after the administration of terbutaline,
monitor closely and be prepared to manage uterine atony and
postpartum hemorrhage

Administration: ritodrine

Obtain laboratory data as ordered (may include CBC, electrolytes,
and glucose)
Place in lateral position during infusion
Monitor maternal ECG as ordered
Administer ritodrine (usually 50 μg/min) via infusion pump or
controller with drug piggybacked into main IV line, being
careful not to exceed maximum dosage of 350 μg/min

Monitor rate and dosage and increase by 50 μg/min q10min based on maternal and fetal responses as ordered

Related patient care

Do not increase dose of terbutaline or ritodrine if patient demonstrates unacceptable side effects: if maternal heart rate exceeds 140 beats/min, if fetal tachycardia of 180 beats/min or greater persists, if systolic blood pressure is <90 mm Hg or more than a 20% decrease, if diastolic BP is <40 mm Hg; do notify physician

Check BP, P, and FHR q10min while increasing dosage, then q30min while patient is receiving IV maintenance dose

Monitor FHR and uterine contractions continuously if possible

Report undesirable side effects, including headache and palpitations, to physician

Continue to maintain IV infusion for 12 hours after arrest of labor, using smallest dose possible to maintain tocolysis

Adjust dosage of tocolytic agent for patients with diurnal patterns of uterine activity

Auscultate lungs q8h to check for fluid overload

Monitor intake and output q1h

Decrease frequency of nursing functions as preterm labor is arrested

Indomethacin (Indocin)
Contraindications

Asthma
Coronary artery disease
Gastrointestinal bleeding (active or past history)
Oligohydramnios
Renal failure
Suspected fetal cardiac or renal anomaly

Assessment

Minimal gastrointestinal disturbance in mother
Fetal effects
    Possible premature closure of patent ductus arteriosus (PDA)
    Possible impaired renal function resulting in oligohydramnios
Neonatal effect
    Temporary decrease in urine output less than 24 hours after last maternal dose
Rare maternal effects—associated with chronic use

Hepatitis
Renal failure
Gastrointestinal bleeding

Administration

Oral administration for **short-term use only** (48 hours)
Initial dose 100-mg rectal suppository followed by 25 mg PO
q6h for 24 to 48 hours
NOTE: Physician may order sucralfate (Carafate) 1 g 30 minutes
before PO doses of indomethacin

Nursing Diagnoses/Interventions/ Evaluation: Preterm Labor

▼Risk for injury to fetus related to potential for preterm delivery; potential for injury to mother related to tocolysis therapy

Maintain bed rest in lateral position; reposition at least q2h
Administer IV fluids as ordered
Note frequency, duration, and strength of contractions q15min and
prn; monitor uterine activity with tocotransducer (tocodyna-
mometer) if available
Auscultate FHR q15min to 30min or electronically monitor with
ultrasound
Measure intake and output as ordered
Assist with amniocentesis and/or ultrasound if ordered
Administer any other medications, including corticosteroids, in ex-
act dose, time, and route as ordered
Decrease frequency of nursing functions as patient's preterm labor
is arrested

If labor continues
See Care of Patient in First Stage of Labor (Appendix E)
In addition
Prepare for high-risk infant
Notify neonatologist or pediatrician
Have resuscitative equipment ready for use
Plan to have infant's blood crossmatched if less than 32
weeks' gestation
Monitor FHR electronically if possible

Assist physician with fetal blood sampling as indicated

Consider plotting labor dilation and descent on square-ruled graph paper (labor is usually rapid, but a high frequency of abnormal labors occur as well, such as Friedman curve)

Provide comfort measures before administering minimal doses of analgesics as ordered

Retain placenta for pathology as ordered

Expected outcome/evaluation

Preterm delivery is avoided; there are no maternal complications of tocolysis therapy

---

▼Risk for situational low self-esteem related to perceptions and expectations of pregnancy and delivery

Encourage patient to verbalize fears and concerns

Note and document

Minimal eye contact

Self-defeating statements and/or behaviors

Overt expressions of guilt or blame

Negativity or inadequacy in actions or verbal communications

Demonstrations of anger

Include significant other in discussions

Provide factual information about placement of blame for initiation and continuation of uterine contractions

Provide positive feedback and encouragement to patient for seeking early interventions

Offer diversional bedrest activities (e.g., reading, TV, computer games, sewing, crossword puzzles, liberal visitation)

Expected outcome/evaluation

Patient verbalizes positive feelings about self

▼Pain related to uterine contractions

Use nonpharmacological measures when appropriate

Positioning

Muscular relaxation techniques

Breathing techniques

Distraction techniques

Eliminate or minimize other factors that could contribute to pain
   Encourage frequent voiding
   Explain all procedures before executing them
   Answer all questions if possible
   Offer choices to allow for control as patient is able
   Keep patient and significant other informed of changes in labor and fetal status
Explain reasons why analgesic agents may not be appropriate
   Effect on FHR
   Possible masking of contractions
   Combined side effects of tocolytic agents and analgesia
Provide positive reinforcement and touch as appropriate
Plan nursing care to provide rest periods to promote comfort, sleep, and relaxation
Assess and document stress-contributing factors to perception of pain
Assess and document q30min
   Frequency and length of contractions
   Location of pain
   Intensity and duration of pain

Expected outcome/evaluation

Patient verbalizes decreasing or more tolerable discomfort

Patient Teaching/Discharge Planning

Explain arrested labor
Emphasize importance of maintaining rest
Emphasize importance of avoiding intercourse, douching, or nipple stimulation, including preparation of breasts for breastfeeding
Teach name of medication, dosage, frequency of administration, purpose, and toxic side effects
Teach or reinforce instructions if patient will be monitored at home with periodic modem transmission of uterine activity
Emphasize importance of having supportive person to perform housekeeping, cooking, and child care tasks
Discuss signs of labor to report to physician
Emphasize importance of follow-up medical care
Discuss development and gestational stage of fetus

Appendix E

Guidelines for Care of the Patient in Labor:
Culturally Sensitive Care
First Stage of Labor
Second and Third Stages of Labor

The following guidelines are for care of the patient during the intrapartum period.* These are basic standards of patient care that can be modified according to institutional policy and practice preferences. This information is included as an adjunct to the care described in Chapter 9, Care of the Monitored Patient.

Guidelines for Culturally Sensitive Obstetrical Patient Care†

Before reviewing the clinical guidelines for care of the patient in labor, the health care provider must focus on the way in which people of different cultures and ethnicities perceive life events, particularly the birthing process, the health care system, and the roles of health care providers. To be effective, patient care must be provided in a culturally sensitive manner.

Self-Assessment

Identify your personal beliefs about persons from cultures different from your own
Review your personal beliefs and past experiences
Set aside any values, biases, ideas, and attitudes that are judgmental and may negatively affect care

*(Modified from Tucker et al: *Patient care standards: collaborative planning and nursing interventions,* ed 7, St Louis, 2000, Mosby.)
†(Modified from Giger J, Davidhizar R: *Transcultural nursing,* ed 3, St Louis, 1999, Mosby.)

258

Patient Assessment

Assess communication variables from a cultural perspective

Determine the ethnic identity of patient, including generation in this country

Use the patient as a source of information when possible

Assess cultural factors that may affect your relationship with the patient and respond appropriately

Interventions

Plan care based on patient's communicated needs and cultural background

Learn as much as possible about patient's cultural customs and beliefs

Encourage patient to reveal cultural interpretation of health, illness, and health care

Be sensitive to the uniqueness of patient

Identify sources of discrepancy between patient's and your own conceptions of health and illness

Communicate at the patient's personal level of functioning

Evaluate effectiveness of patient care actions and modify care plan when necessary

Modify communication approaches to meet cultural needs

Be attentive to signs of fear, anxiety, and confusion

Respond in a reassuring manner in keeping with the patient's cultural orientation

Be aware that in some cultural groups discussion concerning the patient with others may offend and impede patient care activities

Understand that respect and communicated needs are central to the therapeutic relationship

Communicate respect by using a kind and attentive approach

Learn how listening is communicated in the patient's culture

Use appropriate active listening techniques

Adopt an attitude of flexibility, respect, and interest to help bridge barriers imposed by culture

Communicate in a nonthreatening manner

Conduct verbal interactions in an unhurried manner

Follow acceptable social and cultural amenities

Ask general questions during the information gathering stage

Be patient with a respondent who gives information that may seem unrelated to the current health problem

Develop a trusting relationship by listening carefully, allowing time, and giving the patient your full attention

Use validating techniques in communication

Be alert for feedback that the patient is not understanding

Do not assume meaning is interpreted without distortion

Be considerate of reluctance to talk when the subject involves the birthing process (e.g., observation of the perineum when pushing, delivery, and repair)

Be aware that in some cultures these matters are not discussed freely with members of the opposite sex or significant others

Adopt special approaches when the patient speaks a different language

Use a caring tone of voice and facial expression to help alleviate the patient's fears

Speak slowly and distinctly, but not loudly

Use gestures, pictures, and play-acting to help the patient understand

Repeat the message using different words

Be alert to words the patient seems to understand and use them frequently

Keep messages simple and repeat them frequently

Avoid using medical terms and abbreviations that the patient may not understand

Use an appropriate language dictionary

Use interpreters to improve communication

Ask the interpreter to translate the message, not just the individual words

Obtain feedback to confirm understanding

Use an interpreter who is culturally sensitive

Provide caregivers with a common cultural background and language if at all possible

Refer to references on cultural variations for general guidelines

Validate information with patient/family and adjust before applying the information to the patient's individualized plan of care

Communicate cultural variation information with members of the multidisciplinary health care team

Adjust patient care to accommodate cultural preferences as much as possible

Involve patient in adjusting environment to meet cultural needs

Obtain consultation from nutritional services to adjust meal plans to accommodate dietary preferences

Maintain flexibility to provide preferred options with regard to laboring position, anesthesia, etc.

Support routines of spiritual practices and those of support persons

Partner with the patient's family/significant others in planning care, provision of care, and education

Involve members of multidisciplinary care team in adjusting activities to meet cultural preferences, as appropriate

Expected outcomes

Patient

Verbalizes feeling understood

Relates that patient care activities were adjusted to accommodate cultural needs as much as possible

Demonstrates satisfaction with health care providers

Experiences a satisfying therapeutic milieu in the health care setting

Patient Care in First Stage of Labor

Physiologic process by which the fetus is expelled from the uterus

early labor: *Dilation of 0 to 4 cm with mild to moderate irregular contractions*

active labor: *Dilation of 4 to 8 cm with moderate to strong regular contractions every 2 to 5 minutes*

transitional labor: *Dilation of 8 cm to complete dilation with strong contractions*

Assessment
Subjective data

Behavior

Surge of energy and activity

Talking frequently

Anxious

Fear of isolation

Objective data

Rupture of membranes (ROM)
Uterine contractions: regular with increasing intensity and frequency
Transitional labor
  Nausea and vomiting
  Hypersensitive abdomen
  Irritability
  Loss of coping mechanisms
  Hiccups and/or belching
  Trembling and/or shaking of legs
  Chilling
  Perspiration
  Rectal pressure
  Urge to push

Diagnostic tests

Baseline laboratory tests
  CBC with differential
  Hgb/Hct
  Rubella screen
  Hepatitis screen
  VDRL serology
  Chemistries
Urinalysis; protein, glucose
Cultures as indicated by history of signs and symptoms
Ultrasound examination as indicated
Electronic fetal heart rate monitoring
Vibroacoustic stimulation test
Score of Biophysical Profile (if done before onset of labor)

Potential complications

Nonreassuring maternal findings
  Fever
  Hypotension or hypertension
  Dehydration
  Circulatory overload
  Hemorrhage
  Severe pain unrelated to contractions
  Supine hypotension syndrome
  Distended bladder

Nonreassuring fetal findings
  Fetal tachycardia: >160 beats/min
  Fetal bradycardia: <110 beats/min
Fetal hyperactivity or hypoactivity
Monitored labor
  Severe variable decelerations: <70 beats/min for more than 60 seconds
  Uncorrectable, repetitive late decelerations of any magnitude
  Decreased or absent variability
  Prolonged deceleration
  Severe bradycardia
  Unstable FHR; sinusoidal pattern
Inadequate uterine relaxation
  Contractions lasting longer than 90 seconds
  Relaxation between contractions less than 30 seconds
  Tachysystole (>4 contractions in 10 minutes); coupling of uterine contractions
Arrest of labor
Meconium-stained amniotic fluid
Foul-smelling amniotic fluid
Intraamniotic infection secondary to prolonged rupture of membranes
Abruptio placentae

Multidisciplinary Management
Therapeutic management

Prenatal chart and previous medical chart ordered to labor and delivery unit
Laboratory tests as indicated
IV fluids as indicated
Analgesia as indicated per patient reference
Preparation for selected/indicated anesthesia by anesthesiologist/ nurse anesthetist
Supportive care to patient and family

Patient Problems—Nursing Diagnosis/Interventions

▼ Risk for injury to mother related to physiological processes of labor

Assist patient to maintain position of comfort
  Encourage ambulation as tolerated if membranes unruptured and or presenting part is well applied to cervix *to avoid prolapse of cord*
  If membranes are ruptured and presenting part is not engaged, patient should be maintained at bed rest in a comfortable position, avoiding supine hypotension
Assess temperature q2h after rupture of membranes
Plot cervical dilation and fetal descent on Friedman graph *to assess progress of labor*
Offer clear liquids as ordered
Encourage frequent voiding and assist patient to bathroom prn if presenting part is well applied to cervix
  Measure intake and output
  Check urine for protein and glucose
Initiate IV with isotonic solution (lactated Ringer's solution, normal saline) if ordered
  Prehydrate with 1000 to 1500 ml of fluid before regional anesthesia
Maintain dosing of prelabor medications as ordered (anticonvulsants, antihypertensives, or methadone)

Expected outcome

Patient experiences no injury related to labor as evidenced by comfort, adequate hydration, absence of hypotensive episodes related to regional anesthesia, absence of distended bladder, and maintenance of prelabor medical status

▼ Pain and anxiety related to lack of information on physiological processes of labor

Nursing interventions during active labor
  Maintain quiet and calm environment
  Avoid conversation during contractions
  Avoid having persons in room who are not directly caring for patient or providing support *to decrease anxiety*

Make sure nurse call light is accessible
Assist with position changes
    Encourage lateral position
Assist with breathing techniques
    Encourage significant other to be involved in support activities
Apply cool compresses to forehead prn
Apply sacral pressure prn during contractions *to relieve discomfort*
    Encourage support person to give back rub and to apply sacral pressure as needed
Change gown and linens prn
Change pad under buttocks prn
Give pain medication as ordered
Assist with administration of local or regional anesthetic
Record vital signs as per protocol
Nursing interventions during transitional labor
    Palpate abdomen very lightly and only as often as necessary if abdomen is hypersensitive
    Prepare for vomiting episodes
    Encourage patient to empty bladder
    Maintain warmth as necessary
    Encourage patient to avoid pushing until cervix completely dilated
        Panting or rapid blowing breathing technique
    Provide reassurance that transition is relatively short compared with other phases of labor
    Accept aggression or other coping behaviors and avoid negative comments
    Focus on patient and support her by using calm voice, touch, and positive reinforcement

Expected outcome

Experiences manageable pain and minimal anxiety as evidenced by verbalization of same
Complies with assistive directions by staff
Has continuing interaction with significant other/family

▼ Altered oral mucous membrane related to mouth breathing

Administer oral hygiene qh and prn between contractions
  Suck on ice chips, wet washcloths, or sour lollipops unless contraindicated
  Rinse mouth with water and/or mouthwash
  Apply petroleum jelly or antichapping lipsticks to dry lips prn

Expected outcome

Patient does not experience disruption in tissue layers of oral cavity

▼ Risk for altered tissue perfusion related to impaired transport of oxygen associated with uterine contractions and/or uteroplacental insufficiency

Nursing interventions
  Note frequency, duration, and strength of contractions according to facility protocols
  Auscultate FHR for 1 minute immediately after uterine contractions in nonelectronically monitored labor
    Every 15 to 30 minutes and prn
  Assess FHR immediately after spontaneous or artificial amniotomy *to assess for prolapsed umbilical cord*
  Assess maternal vital signs per institutional protocol
    T, P, and R every 2 to 4 hours and prn
    BP and P q2h and prn
  Initiate intrauterine resuscitation protocols for nonreassuring fetal findings as indicated
    Turn mother to lateral position
    Increase rate of isotonic IV solution
    Administer 100% oxygen by snug face mask at 8 to 10 L/min
    Notify physician of situation

Expected outcome

Patient gives birth to newborn in good condition with Apgar score ≥8 at 5 minutes of age

Patient/Family Teaching

Allay anxiety as much as possible by doing the following
  Explain reasons for performing all procedures

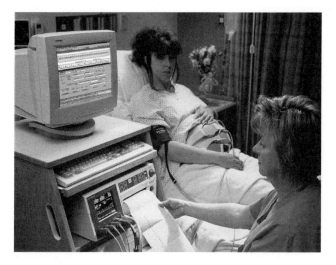

Figure E-1
Monitoring the patient in labor with a twin gestation.
(Courtesy GE Marquette Medical Systems, Milwaukee, Wis.)

Encourage spouse or significant other to remain with patient to provide support during labor

Assist spouse or significant other to listen to fetal heart with fetoscope, Doppler, or ultrasound equipment

Provide supportive care based on patient's and family's knowledge of labor process

Ask patient if she wants additional support persons present for labor and birth

Inform waiting family and friends about patient's progress and inform patient that they are waiting and interested

Reduce environmental stimuli that may contribute to anxiety and tension; provide relaxed, restful atmosphere

Reassure patient at appropriate intervals that labor is progressing and that both patient and fetus are doing well

Procedural Care of Patient During Delivery: Second and Third Stages of Labor

The stage of expulsion of the fetus, placenta, and membranes after complete dilatation of the cervix

Assessment
Subjective data

Extreme anxiety
Patient stating, "Baby is coming"
Desire to defecate
Fear of losing control

Objective data

Involuntary bearing down/pushing
Grunting sounds
Vomiting
Involuntary shaking of thighs
Perspiration between nose and upper lip
Increase in bloody show
Prolonged second stage
   More than 1 hour for multigravidas
   More than 2 hours for primigravidas
Crowning

Diagnostic tests

Electronic fetal monitoring
Cord blood: gases, pH, and other tests as ordered

Potential complications

Fetal stress/distress
Birth asphyxia
Difficult birth
   Cephalopelvic disproportion
   Shoulder dystocia
   Breech presentation
Forceps delivery
Vacuum extraction
Cesarean birth
Infant bruising, fractures

Nursing management
Care during delivery

Auscultate FHR q5min and/or after each push if electronic monitor is not used (if electronic monitor was used continuously during labor, then it should be continued in the delivery room until the time of delivery)

Check BP and P q10min and prn

Pad stirrups or foot/leg supports if used

Administer oxygen mask at 8 to 10 L/min as ordered

Understand that low- to semi-Fowler's position with lateral tilt is preferred while pushing

Assist with breathing techniques

Deep ventilation before and after each contraction

Open-glottis breathing when pushing with contractions

Observe perineum while pushing

Notify physician if second stage is prolonged

Prepare perineum according to hospital procedure

Place nurse, spouse, and/or labor coach at head of delivery table to encourage patient during delivery process

Encourage long, sustained pushing rather than frequent short pushes

Encourage patient to push when she feels urge to push

Work with patient to find a rhythm for pushing that is most effective for her

Encourage complete relaxation between contractions

Reassure patient that she is doing well and is advancing fetus with each push

Apply cool, moist cloth to forehead as needed

Keep DeLee suction catheter available and ready to use if meconium-stained amniotic fluid is present

Plan for suctioning of naso-oropharynx after delivery of fetal head and before delivery of thorax to prevent meconium aspiration

Have resuscitation equipment and Neonatal Resuscitation Program (NRP) trained personnel ready for delivery

Assist physician or nurse-midwife as needed

Immediate postpartum care (fourth-stage care)

Encourage mother to inspect infant as soon as possible

Place infant on maternal abdomen to provide skin-to-skin contact if delivery room is warm

Defer neonatal eye therapy for 1 to 2 hours after birth to promote eye contact with mother; administer eye therapy per hospital policy

Assess BP and P q10min to 15min × 4 and prn

Add oxytocic drug as ordered to parenteral fluids

Palpate fundus for tone several times in the first 2 hours after delivery (e.g., q15min × 4, then q30min × 2 or 5min to 10min × 4 and prn)

Assess maternal BP and P frequently during the first 2 hours after delivery (e.g., q15min × 4, then q30min × 2 or q10min to 15min × 4 and prn)

Administer perineal care before removing legs from stirrups *to cleanse and inspect perineum*

Place sterile perineal pad under buttocks before transporting patient to recovery area

Place ice pack on episiotomy unless otherwise ordered *to reduce swelling*

Assist with infant's warm water bath if newborn's temperature is stable

Maintain mother's warmth with blankets as needed

Place radiant heat warmer over upper part of mother's bed or place dry, warmly blanketed newborn next to mother *so that she can visually inspect, touch, and/or breast-feed nude infant while preventing neonatal heat loss*

Encourage mother and spouse and/or labor coach to be with infant in delivery area, providing them with as much privacy as feasible unless this is contraindicated by maternal or neonatal pathological condition

Encourage mother to freely express her feelings about herself and her infant

Explain that behaviors manifested in labor are normal and there is no reason to be embarrassed, if mother is apologetic for behavior

Appendix F

Selected Pattern Interpretation at 3 Centimeters per Minute Paper Speed

The paper speed used in the following tracings is 3 cm/min. This speed is commonly used in North America for paper that is scaled from 30 to 240 bpm.

External Mode of Monitoring— Interpretable Tracing

SIGNAL SOURCE   Ultrasound and tocotransducer

FHR   Baseline: 140 bpm

    Variability: Moderate

    Periodic changes: No significant changes

UTERINE ACTIVITY   Frequency: 2 to 2½ minutes

    Duration: 30 to 50 seconds

Note the zigzag maternal respiratory movements of the uterine activity panel.

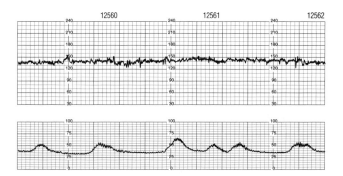

Loose Spiral Electrode With Complete Cervical Dilation

SIGNAL SOURCE

Spiral electrode and tocotransducer

FHR

Baseline: 136 bpm in panel 55986. The sudden loss of FHR signal in panel 55987 is due to a loose spiral electrode (lead), because complete dilatation has occurred. The actual FHR was then auscultated at 136 bpm, which is consistent with the previously known baseline.

Variability: Unable to determine

Periodic changes: Unable to determine

UTERINE ACTIVITY

Frequency: 2½ to 3 minutes

Duration: 50 to 90 seconds

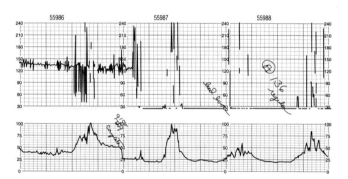

Uterine Tachysystole With Hypertonus

SIGNAL SOURCE	Ultrasound and tocotransducer
FHR	Baseline: 120-130 bpm
	Variability: Moderate
	Nonperiodic changes: Initially an acceleration is present
UTERINE ACTIVITY	Tachysystole (increased number of contractions) and poor relaxation between contractions
	Frequency: 1 to 1½ minutes
	Duration: 40 to 50 seconds

This patient had a transverse lie, the cervix was undilated, and she was delivered by primary cesarean for a suspected (then confirmed) placental abruption.

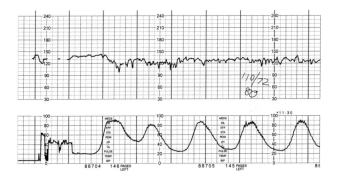

Coupling of Uterine Contractions

SIGNAL SOURCE   Spiral electrode and intrauterine catheter

FHR   Baseline: 130 bpm

                    Variability: Moderate

                    Periodic changes: No significant changes

UTERINE ACTIVITY   Frequency: 1½ to 4½ minutes

                    Duration: 40 seconds

                    Intensity: 60 mm Hg

                    Resting tone: 5 mm Hg

Laboring patterns vary among individuals. Note the characteristic coupling of uterine contractions in this tracing.

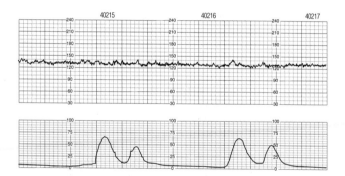

Early Decelerations

SIGNAL SOURCE	Ultrasound and tocotransducer
FHR	Baseline: 120 bpm
	Variability: Not specific with ultrasound but probably minimal
	Periodic changes: Consistent early decelerations occur with each contraction because of head compression.
UTERINE ACTIVITY	Frequency: 2 to 3 minutes
	Duration: 40 to 50 seconds

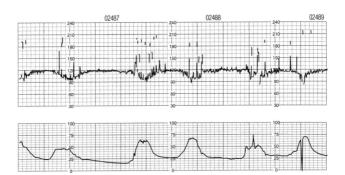

Acceleration of Fetal Heart Rate With Uterine Contractions

SIGNAL SOURCE	Spiral electrode and intrauterine catheter
FHR	Baseline: 130 bpm
	Variability: Moderate
	Periodic changes: Acceleration of FHR occurs with each contraction and with fetal movement as evidenced by the spikes in the UA panel just before the two middle contractions. Sometimes acceleration of FHR with contractions or before contractions makes the FHR look as if late decelerations are occurring, when given a casual glance. Therefore it is important to identify the baseline rate and note the timing of the acceleration or deceleration in relation to the uterine contraction.
UTERINE ACTIVITY	Frequency: 3 to 3½ minutes
	Duration: 60 to 70 seconds
	Intensity: Probably 75 to 85 mm Hg
	Resting tone: Probably 30 to 35 mm Hg

The UA section was not zeroed before use. The resting tone and intensity of the contractions are most likely much lower than are reflected in this tracing.

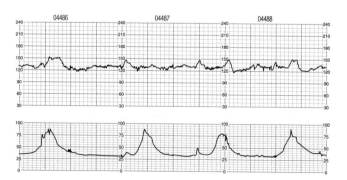

Acceleration of Fetal Heart Rate With Uterine Contraction

SIGNAL SOURCE Spiral electrode and tocotransducer

FHR   Baseline: 140 to 150 bpm

        Variability: Moderate

        Periodic changes: Acceleration of FHR occurs with each contraction. The amplitude of the acceleration is markedly increased when the patient pushes with contractions.

UTERINE ACTIVITY Frequency: 2½ minutes

        Duration: 40 to 50 seconds

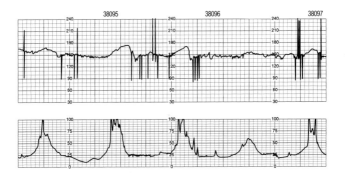

Variable Decelerations

SIGNAL SOURCE	Spiral electrode and tocotransducer
FHR	Baseline: 140 bpm
	Variability: Moderate
	Nonperiodic changes: Mild variable decelerations in FHR occur with each contraction. This frequently occurs with pushing and signals the second stage of labor.
UTERINE ACTIVITY	Frequency: 1½ to 2 minutes
	Duration: 30 to 40 seconds

Spikes of uterine pressure above 50 mm Hg indicate maternal pushing.

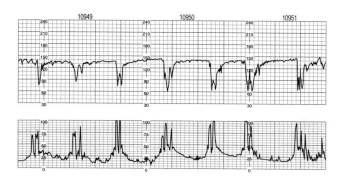

Variable Decelerations

SIGNAL SOURCE	Spiral electrode and IUPC
FHR	Baseline: 150 to 160 bpm
	Variability: Moderate
	Nonperiodic changes: Variable decelerations, shoulders, and "overshoots" are evidenced
UTERINE ACTIVITY	Frequency: 1½ to 3 minutes
	Duration: 50 to 60 seconds
	Intensity: 60 mm Hg
	Resting tone: 10 to 20 mm Hg

This tracing demonstrates a variety of periodic variable decelerations that become more significant as labor progresses.

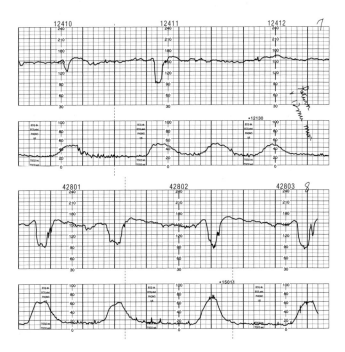

Prolonged Deceleration/Variable Decelerations—Uterine Rupture

SIGNAL SOURCE	Spiral electrode and IUPC
FHR	Baseline: 140 to 150 bpm
	Variability: Moderate LTV, present STV
	Nonperiodic changes: Prolonged deceleration, variable decelerations
UTERINE ACTIVITY	Frequency: 2 to 2½ minutes
	Duration: 30 to 40 seconds
	Intensity: 30 to 40 mm Hg
	Resting tone: 10 to 15 mm Hg

The tracings previous to this one were all reassuring. At the time of the uterine rupture, the prolonged deceleration was evidenced. The FHR then returned to its baseline and variables were noted. The variables increased in duration and became more significant, and the baseline FHR increased to a tachycardic level in a very short period. The decelerations also took on a late component with a decrease in variability.

Upon delivery, the entire old scar from a previous cesarean ruptured and the rupture extended into the cervix. A hysterectomy was not required, but an extensive repair was needed. The infant's Apgars were 8 at 1 minute and 9 at 5 minutes.

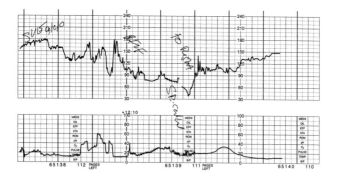

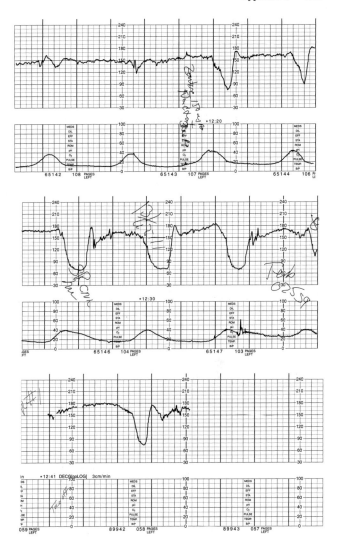

Variable Decelerations/Prolapsed Umbilical Cord

SIGNAL SOURCE | Spiral electrode and tocotransducer

FHR | Baseline: Unable to establish; perhaps 150 to 160 bpm

Variability: Moderate LTV, present STV

Nonperiodic change: Prolonged decelerations resulting from umbilical cord prolapse

UTERINE CONTRACTIONS | It is probable that there are contractions within this segment that do not record. Perhaps in the haste to intervene when this pattern occurred, the tocotransducer was removed.

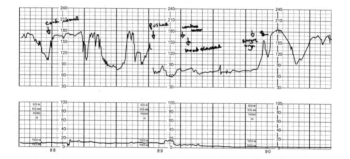

Fetal Tachycardia

SIGNAL SOURCE	Spiral electrode and tocotransducer
FHR	Baseline: 190 to 200 bpm
	Variability: Moderate
	Periodic changes: No significant changes; a mild variable deceleration occurs in panel 30266.
UTERINE ACTIVITY	Frequency: 2 to 2½ minutes
	Duration: 30 to 40 seconds

Note the wide-excursion vertical lines, probably caused by electrical "noise" or interference. If these lines were more frequent and consistent, they would suggest a fetal arrhythmia.

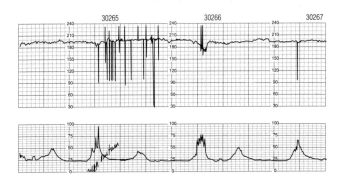

Minimal Variability

SIGNAL SOURCE	Spiral electrode and tocotransducer
FHR	Baseline: 140 to 150 bpm
	Variability: Minimal
	Periodic changes: No significant changes
UTERINE ACTIVITY	Either contractions are not present or the tocotransducer is misplaced. The uterine activity demonstrated here is normal for the patient who is not in labor. Maternal respiratory movements are clearly seen.

This fetus was 3 weeks overdue and later delivered spontaneously with a meconium-stained placenta, birth weight of 4067 g (9 lb 1¼ oz), and Apgar scores of 4 at 1 minute and 7 at 5 minutes of age.

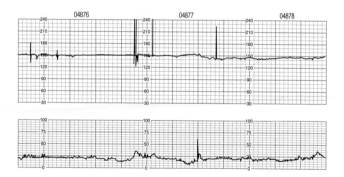

Sine Wave (Pseudosinusoidal) or Undulating Pattern

SIGNAL SOURCE   Ultrasound and tocotransducer

FHR   Baseline: 120 to 140 bpm

                       Variability: Moderate

                       Periodic changes: None

UTERINE ACTIVITY   None

   Sine wave in this instance is benign. A true sinusoidal pattern is characterized by extreme regularity and smoothness. Although narcotics may cause this type of sine wave, they were not the cause in this case. Some experts think that fetal sucking or mouthing motions will cause this pattern (van Woerden, 1988; Nijhuis, 1984). It is often preceded or followed by a period of accelerations. In this case, that was true. In the next 10-minute window, the baseline was noted at 120 to 130 bpm and accelerations were apparent.

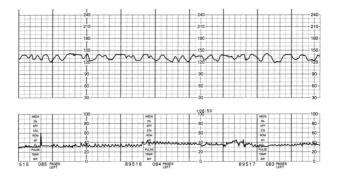

Sinusoidal Pattern

SIGNAL SOURCE	Spiral electrode and intrauterine pressure catheter
FHR	Baseline: 140 to 150 bpm
	Variability: Sinusoidal pattern with undulating sine wave
	Periodic changes: None

Note that the sinusoidal pattern is characterized by regularity and smoothness

UTERINE ACTIVITY   Not in active labor

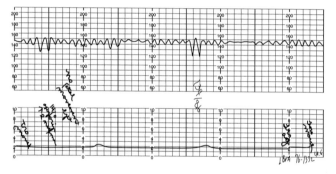

Figure F-15
(Courtesy Roger K. Freeman, MD, Long Beach, Calif.)

Fetal Cardiac Arrhythmia

SIGNAL SOURCE	Spiral electrode and intrauterine catheter
FHR	Baseline: 170 bpm; the vertical excursions from the baseline indicate a cardiac arrhythmia. If they were less frequent and more random, they would suggest electrical interference or "noise." Clinically, this pattern is not a cause for consideration of termination of labor. Most fetal cardiac arrhythmias disappear after birth and are not considered a sign of fetal distress.
	Variability: Minimal
UTERINE ACTIVITY	Frequency: 1½ to 6 minutes
	Duration: 50 to 60 seconds
	Intensity: 50+ mm Hg with patient pushing
	Resting tone: 10 mm Hg

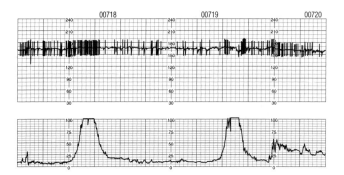

Lambda Pattern

SIGNAL SOURCE	Ultrasound and tocotransducer
FHR	Baseline: 128 to 140 bpm
	Variability: Average
	Periodic changes: Acceleration
UTERINE ACTIVITY	One contraction noted
	Duration: 70 seconds
	Intensity: By palpation, mild

The lambda pattern is one that is common in early labor. It consists of an acceleration followed by a deceleration and then returns to baseline. The pattern is associated with uterine contractions. Typically appearing in early labor, this pattern does not persist (Freeman, Garite, Nageotte, 1991) and its physiology is unknown. It is included because it does occur and should not be confused with a late deceleration or other nonreassuring patterns.

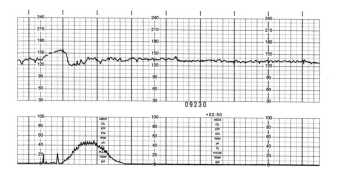

Interesting Pattern

Gravida 1 at term induced for pregnancy-induced hypertension; artificial rupture of membranes after admission with meconium-stained fluid and amnioinfusion begun. There is no information on the tracing with regard to changes in the infusion rate of oxytocin. Epidural was placed, with redoses q60min to 90min in spite of pump being used. Note maternal vital signs throughout tracing. The time on the monitor strip is the correct time (the Dinamap time is incorrect). Although the patient was continuously monitored, only selected sections are included for interest. The intervening pattern looked the same as the panels preceding and following the displayed panels.

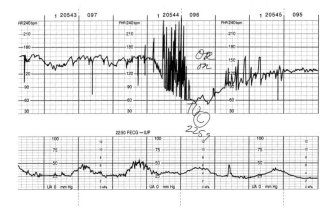

Panel 20544: Patient's epidural was redosed and there was a prolonged deceleration. Patient was turned and oxygen given.

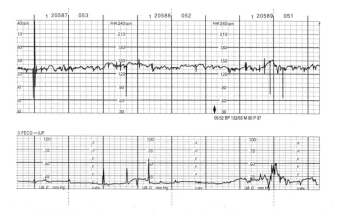

Panel 20588: FHR exhibits moderate (average) variability and normal baseline rate. The IUPC was replaced shortly after the end of panel 20589 and before the tracing on p. 289.

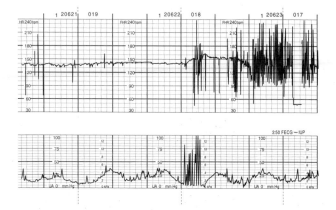

Panel 20623: Patient was agitated, with nausea, vomiting, and complaints of "numbness" (location unspecified). Note spikes in uterine activity panel indicative of vomiting.

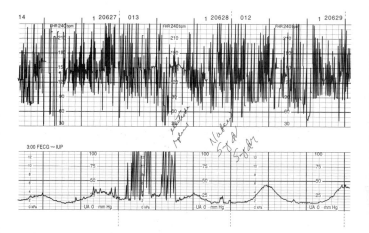

Panel 20628: The electrode was replaced, and the patient was given Nubain 5 mg IV and 5 mg IM.

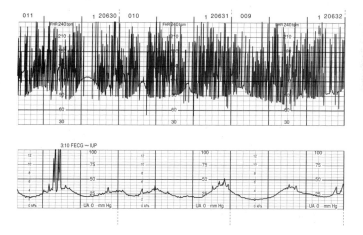

Panel 20630: The physician was requested to evaluate the patient about 3:10 AM.

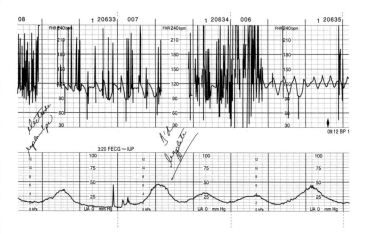

Panel 20633-34: A new spiral electrode and leg plate were placed. The contractions are less than 1½ minutes apart.

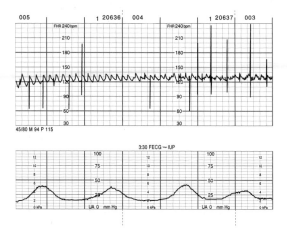

Panel 20635: The pattern becomes clearer and appears initially to be similar to a *checkmark* pattern indicative of fetal seizure activity (Freeman, Garite, Nageotte, 1991); however, the appearance of the pattern changes in **panel 20637** and appears to be similar to patterns associated with cardiac arrhythmias. It would have been interesting to view a concurrent fetal ECG. Note the diminishing amplitude of the baseline FHR.

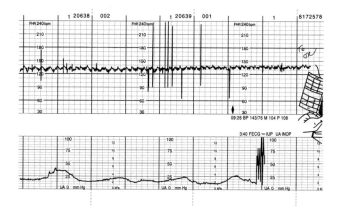

Panel 20638: The pattern continues, with diminishing amplitude.

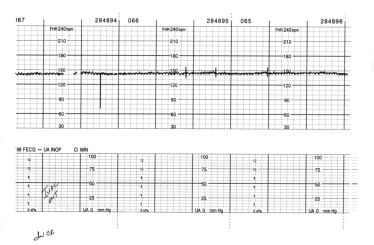

Panel 28494: The patient has been moved to the operating room (and connected to another monitor), and the baseline is becoming flatter.

The Apgars are unknown; however, the cord pH was 6.9 and the neonate did not have good respiratory effort. The neonate was placed on a ventilator and transported to a tertiary center and was off the ventilator ≤48 hours. Additional information and any sequelae are unknown.

Appendix G

Clinical Competencies and Education Guide: Antepartum and Intrapartum Fetal Heart Rate Monitoring

Preface
Framework for Practice

The use of electronic and manual devices to assess the fetal heart rate in the antepartum and intrapartum settings has long been a practice of obstetric nurses. The purpose of this document is to describe the guidelines for the core content of educational programs and clinical practicums for fetal heart rate monitoring. This document outlines specific areas of proficiency required of each nurse whose practice includes the use of antepartum and intrapartum fetal heart rate monitoring. Actual achievement of competency depends upon individual skills, training and clinical experience.

Introduction
Nursing Competency

In this document, *competent* is defined as having requisite qualities, capacity or ability. *Competence,* with respect to antepartum and intrapartum fetal heart rate monitoring, means having and being able to use a core knowledge base regarding electronic fetal heart monitoring and auscultation. Participation in a formal program of instruction and clinical practicum are necessary to achieve competent performance.

This document presents a suggested framework for didactic in-

Used by permission of Association of Women's Health, Obstetric and Neonatal Nurses (1998); 2000 L St., NW, Suite 740, Washington, DC 20036, 1-800-673-8499 (US) or 1-800-245-0231 (Canada) http://www.awhonn.org

struction and includes a variety of clinical practicum opportunities from which individual institutions may draw. This open-ended approach is necessitated by the fact that no data exist to support one "best" way to prepare for or evaluate an individual nurse's clinical competence in antepartum and intrapartum fetal heart rate monitoring.

Didactic Instruction

Didactic instruction, for the purpose of this document, is defined as the intentional and planned act or practice that has the goal of imparting knowledge or a lesson. Didactic instruction should be grounded in evidence-based research and can be presented through various learning modalities. These modalities include, but are not limited to, classroom lectures, self-programmed instruction, textbooks, instructional videotapes, and computer assisted learning programs.

Clinical Learning Experiences or Practicums

A *clinical practicum* is defined for the purpose of this document as a supervised, repeated performance of an activity or skill set for the purpose of learning or perfecting a skill. The individual responsible for the supervision of the task may be referred to as a clinical instructor, preceptor, or trainer. A qualified instructor may be a professional nurse or physician who has prior demonstration of competency in the activity or skill set. Clinical learning experiences or practicums may be supervised by more than one individual.

Antepartum Fetal Heart Rate Monitoring
Nursing Practice Competencies

1. Describe the technical basis of EFM and correctly use and troubleshoot the technology
2. Describe antepartum testing criteria, indications for testing and use of appropriate test results
3. Communicate the physiologic premise for each test, and discuss fetal outcomes based on test results
4. Recognize the indications and contraindications for each test
5. Provide patient education regarding the procedure and its purpose

6. Demonstrate skill in electronic fetal monitoring:
   a. Turn the monitor on, adjust individual features of the monitor (e.g., clock and arrhythmia filter activation) and test the machine for internal calibration
   b. Correctly refill tracing paper and check paper speed
   c. Perform abdominal palpation to determine fetal position and the appropriate site for fetal heart rate (FHR) ultrasound transducer placement
   d. Perform abdominal palpation to determine the location of the uterine fundus for tocodynamometer (TOCO) external transducers and adjust the electronic fetal monitor accordingly
   e. Identify technically inadequate tracing and take appropriate corrective action
   f. Obtain and maintain an adequate tracing of the fetal heart and uterine contractions; use troubleshooting techniques to check accuracy of signal acquisition (ultrasound transducer function)
   g. Assess uterine contraction frequency and duration, palpate for contraction intensity and baseline resting tone; determine whether normal or abnormal findings are present
   h. Identify baseline fetal heart rate and presence of periodic and nonperiodic changes
7. Conduct the prescribed antepartum test and interpret test results
8. Implement intervention per institutional protocol when indicated
9. Communicate the content and interpretation of antepartum test results in written and verbal form in accordance with institutional guidelines
10. Discontinue electronic fetal monitoring according to institutional guidelines
11. Communicate and document appropriate follow-up information to the patient
12. Demonstrate maintenance of electronic fetal monitoring equipment.

Didactic Content Outline

I. Elements of antepartum fetal heart monitoring
   A. Goals of antepartum fetal heart monitoring

        b. Techniques

        c. Sources of error and limitations

        d. Advantages and disadvantages

      2. External electronic: tocodynamometer

        a. Technical principles

        b. Application and nursing care during use

        c. Sources of error and limitations

        d. Advantages and disadvantages

    B. Fetal heart rate monitoring

      1. External electronic: ultrasound transducer

        a. Principles of Doppler ultrasound

        b. Application and care during use

        c. Sources of error and limitations

        d. Advantages and disadvantages

V. Interpretation of antepartum fetal monitoring

    A. Nonstress test

      1. Definition of test

      2. Physiologic basis of test

      3. Test procedure

      4. Interpretation of test results

      5. Patient education

      6. Follow up

    B. Contraction stress test

      1. Definition of test

      2. Physiologic basis of test

      3. Test procedure: exogenous or endogenous

        a. Nipple stimulation

        b. Oxytocin

      4. Contraindications for the contraction stress test

      5. Interpretation of test results

      6. Patient education

      7. Follow up

Clinical Learning Experiences and Evaluation

The sequence and specific nature of clinical learning experiences can be adapted to accommodate the style of the clinical instructor/ preceptor and the needs of the individual learner.

    Practice sessions may include:

1. Review of evidence-based policies, procedures and protocols
2. Electronic fetal monitor tracing review sessions
3. Small group discussion/case studies

4. Clinical conferences (multidisciplinary when possible)
5. Role-play situations
6. Videotaped observation and follow-up discussion
7. Computer simulation
8. One-to-one tutorial
9. Programmed self-study
10. Simulation with models for skill practice

Learner Assessment

Validation of ability to function independently evolves as a process through the didactic and clinical learning period. Instructor/preceptor evaluation and self-evaluation should be ongoing during the training period and conducted periodically once independent nursing practice is initiated. Evaluation of performance ability may include the following:

1. Verbal or written exercises, such as
   a. Examination
   b. Case study analysis
   c. Electronic fetal monitor tracing interpretation sessions
   d. Identification of the institution's policies, procedures and protocols
   e. Identification of lines of authority and responsibility (chain of command)
   f. Verbal and written communication of findings
   g. Ability to initiate conflict resolution
2. Observation by instructor/preceptor of nurse providing patient care in fetal heart monitor clinical situations.

Intrapartum Fetal Heart Rate Monitoring
Nursing Practice Competencies

1. Implement the appropriate fetal heart monitoring method based on primary care provider order, patient status, patient request, hospital policy, unit staffing resources and current standards of practice recommended by professional organizations
2. Explain the principles of the chosen method of fetal heart monitoring to the patient and her support person(s)
3. Identify the limitations of information produced by each method of monitoring

4. Demonstrate skill in fetal heart monitoring by auscultation
    a. Perform abdominal palpation to determine fetal position and the appropriate site for fetoscope and/or Doppler placement
    b. Apply a fetoscope or Doppler device to the selected site
    c. Palpate uterine contractions for frequency, duration and intensity; assess resting tone between contractions; determine whether abnormal findings are present
    d. Identify the baseline fetal heart rate and rhythm and their relationship to the uterine contraction
    e. Interpret the findings and implement nursing interventions
    f. Identify the clinical situations, based on fetal monitoring findings, in which immediate notification of the primary health care provider is indicated
    g. Communicate the findings to the primary care provider(s) and the patient
    h. Document entries on the written or computerized patient record
    i. Demonstrate skill in maintenance and troubleshooting of auscultation equipment
5. Demonstrate skill in continuous electronic fetal monitoring
    a. Turn the monitor on, adjust individual features of the monitor (e.g., clock, arrhythmia filter activation), test the machine for internal calibration, refill tracing paper and check paper speed
    b. Perform abdominal palpation to determine fetal position and the appropriate site for FHR ultrasound transducer placement
    c. Perform abdominal palpation to determine the location of the uterine fundus for TOCO transducer placement
    d. Apply both the FHR and TOCO external transducers and adjust the electronic fetal monitor accordingly
    e. Prepare the patient, set up equipment and correctly apply the internal fetal spiral electrode (when the individual's training, state and/or provincial nurse practice act and hospital policy allow)
    f. Prepare the patient, set up equipment and insert an intrauterine pressure catheter (when the individual's training, state and/or provincial nurse practice acts and hospital policy allow)

g. Zero the monitor for use with an intrauterine pressure catheter

h. Identify technically inadequate tracings and take appropriate corrective action

i. Obtain and maintain an adequate tracing of the fetal heart and uterine contractions; use troubleshooting techniques to check accuracy of signal acquisition (ultrasound transducer function, fetal spiral electrode leg plate test and intrauterine pressure catheter testing procedures)

j. Assess uterine contraction frequency, duration, intensity and baseline resting tone as appropriate based on monitoring method and determine whether normal or abnormal findings are present

k. Identify baseline fetal heart rate and rhythm, variability and the presence of periodic and nonperiodic changes

l. Classify the findings and implement appropriate nursing interventions

m. Discuss findings with the patient and support person(s)

n. Identify the clinical situations, based on EFM findings, in which immediate notification of the primary health care provider is indicated

o. Communicate the content of electronic fetal monitoring data, interpretation of data, resulting nursing interventions and outcome of interventions in written and verbal form

p. Document entries in the written or computerized patient record on the electronic fetal monitoring tracing or in the fetal monitor data storage and retrieval system

q. Demonstrate maintenance of electronic fetal monitoring equipment.

Didactic Content Outline

I. Elements in fetal heart rate monitoring
   A. Goals of fetal heart rate monitoring
      1. Determine fetal heart rate characteristics and uterine activity
      2. Assess fetal well-being and tolerance to labor

B. Methods of monitoring
   1. Intermittent auscultation
     a. Fetoscope
     b. Doppler ultrasound
   2. Electronic fetal monitoring
     a. External
     b. Internal
   3. Selection of method/combination of methods

II. Physiologic basis for interpretation
  A. Origin of the fetal heart rate
    1. Physiology of the fetal cardiac conduction system
    2. Parasympathetic innervation
    3. Sympathetic innervation
    4. Chemoreceptor influences
    5. Baroreceptor influences
    6. Humoral influences
  B. Physiology of fetal gas exchange
    1. Maternal uteroplacental circulation
    2. Maternal arterial blood gas
    3. Fetal umbilical placental circulation
    4. Fetal arterial blood gas
  C. Pathophysiology of fetal gas exchange
    1. Maternal factors
      a. Impaired circulation
      b. Impaired oxygen exchange
    2. Uterine contractions
      a. Endogenous causes
      b. Exogenous causes
    3. Placental factors
      a. Impaired circulation
      b. Impaired oxygen exchange
    4. Umbilical cord factors
      a. Compression
      b. Occlusion
      c. Compromised perfusion
    5. Fetal factors
      a. Impaired circulation
      b. Impaired oxygen exchange

III. Physiologic principles of uterine activity
  A. Physiology of uterine contractions and resting tone

B. Normal alterations in fetal oxygenation related to uterine activity

C. Abnormal alterations in fetal oxygenation related to uterine activity

IV. Monitoring techniques

   A. Uterine activity monitoring

     1. Palpation

       a. Principles

       b. Techniques

       c. Sources of error and limitations

       d. Advantages and disadvantages

     2. External electronic: tocodynamometer

       a. Technical principles

       b. Application and nursing care during use

       c. Sources of error and limitations

       d. Advantages and disadvantages

     3. Internal electronic: intrauterine pressure catheter

       a. Types and technical principles

         (1) Fluid-filled catheters

         (2) Transducer-tipped catheters

       b. Application and care during use

       c. Calibration of monitor

       d. Zeroing the transducer

       e. Sources of error and limitations

       f. Advantages and disadvantages

   B. Fetal heart rate

     1. External auscultation

       a. Types and technical principles

         (1) Fetoscope

         (2) Doppler ultrasound

       b. Techniques of signal acquisition

       c. Sources of error and limitations

       d. Advantages and disadvantages

     2. External electronic: ultrasound transducer

       a. Principles of Doppler ultrasound

       b. Application and care during use

       c. Sources of error and limitations

       d. Advantages and disadvantages

     3. Internal electronic: fetal spiral electrode

       a. Principles of cardiotachometry

          4. Contraction intensity
             a. Assessment guidelines
             b. Limitations
      B. Uterine activity: internal intrauterine pressure catheter
          1. Resting tone
          2. Contraction frequency
          3. Contraction duration
          4. Contraction intensity
  VIII. Interpretation of electronic fetal heart rate by continuous EFM
      A. Baseline fetal heart rate and rhythm
          1. Definition
          2. Physiologic basis of baseline rate(s)
          3. Normal range
             a. Full-term
             b. Effect of gestational age
          4. Tachycardia
             a. Definition
             b. Clinical significance
             c. Interventions
          5. Bradycardia
             a. Definition
             b. Clinical significance
             c. Interventions
          6. Dysrhythmia/Arrhythmia
             a. Definition
             b. Clinical significance
             c. Interventions
          7. Sinusoidal
             a. Definition
             b. Clinical significance
             c. Interventions
          8. Variability
             a. Physiologic mechanism
             b. Interpretation
             c. Clinical significance
             d. Interventions
      B. Periodic fetal heart rate patterns
          1. Accelerations
             a. Definition

C. Planning and intervention
   1. Independent nursing actions based on interpreted data
   2. Fetal heart monitoring findings necessitating immediate notification of primary health care provider
   3. Documentation
D. Evaluation
   1. Response to intervention
   2. Documentation
   3. Altering plan of nursing care based on response to intervention

Clinical Learning Experiences and Evaluations

The sequence and specific nature of clinical learning experiences can be adapted to accommodate the style of the clinical instructor/preceptor and the needs of the individual learner.

Practice sessions may include:

1. Review of evidence-based policy, procedures and protocols
2. Electronic fetal monitor tracing review sessions
3. Auscultated heart rate review sessions
4. Small group discussions/case studies
5. Clinical conferences (multidisciplinary when possible)
6. Role-play situations
7. Videotaped observation and follow-up discussion
8. Computer simulation
9. One-to-one tutorial
10. Programmed self-study
11. Simulation with models for skill practice

Learner Assessment

Validation of ability to function independently evolves as a process through the didactic and clinical learning period. Instructor/preceptor evaluation and self-evaluation should be ongoing during the training period and conducted periodically once independent nursing practice is initiated. Evaluation of ability may include the following:

1. Verbal or written exercises, such as:
   a. Examination
   b. Case study analysis

c. Electronic fetal monitoring tracing interpretation sessions
d. Auscultated fetal heart rate interpretation sessions
e. Identification of the institution's policies, procedures and protocols
f. Identification of lines of authority and responsibility (chain of command)
g. Verbal and written communication of findings
h. Ability to initiate conflict resolution
2. Observation by instructor/preceptor of nurse providing patient care in fetal heart monitor clinical situations

Ongoing Competency Validation

No agreed upon method exists to enhance or measure ongoing competency of professional nursing practice. Additionally, data do not exist to define the impact of current competency validation of fetal heart rate monitoring on patient outcomes. Therefore, maintaining the quality of individual practice in accordance with current guidelines and standards requires the exercise of judgment and responsibility by institutions and the professional nurse.

Summary

It is estimated that fetal heart rate monitoring (by either auscultation or EFM) can reduce the intrapartum fetal death rate from 1.76/1,000 births to .5/1,000 births (ACOG, 1995). Unfortunately, neither method of intrapartum monitoring is effective in preventing or predicting long-term neurologic outcomes. Choice of fetal monitoring techniques should be a collaborative and informed decision between the patient and her primary care provider. Regardless of the method of fetal monitoring chosen, evidence supports the need for a one-to-one nurse patient ratio for women in active labor. Hodnett's (1997) meta-analysis of trials of labor support concludes that the presence of a trained support person reduces the likelihood of medication for pain relief, operative vaginal birth, cesarean birth and a 5-minute Apgar score less than 7.

This document provides guidelines for educational preparation that provide a foundation for appropriate performance of antepartum and intrapartum fetal heart rate monitoring. The performance of fetal monitoring in obstetric nursing practice requires formal education, including theoretical content and hands-on experience by obstetric professionals. Nurses can perform fetal monitoring in accordance with their training and according to institutional policy, state and provincial practice acts, if such procedures are within their scope of practice. These guidelines were generated in response to nurses seeking direction in the design of fetal heart rate monitoring educational programs. This document provides recommendations and suggestions for programs to assist nurses obtaining appropriate training to perform antepartum and intrapartum fetal heart rate monitoring. The task force encourages nurses and institutions to continue additional training, education and competency assessment programs and to evaluate patient outcomes that are based on the proficiency level of the nursing care providers.

References

Albers, L.L. (1994). Clinical issues in electronic fetal monitoring. *Birth, 21,* 108-110.

American Academy of Pediatrics and American College of Obstetricians and Gynecologists. (1997). *Guidelines for perinatal care* (4th ed.). Elk Grove Village, IL: Author.

American College of Obstetricians and Gynecologists (1995). *Fetal heart rate patterns: Monitoring, interpretation and management.* (Technical Bulletin 207). Washington, D.C.: Author.

Association of Women's Health, Obstetric and Neonatal Nurses. (1998). *Clinical competencies and education guide: Limited ultrasound examinations in obstetric and gynecologic/infertility settings.* Washington DC: Author.

Davies, B.L., Niday, P.A., Nimrod, C.A., Drake, E.R., Sprague, A.E., & Trepanier, M.J. (1993). Electronic fetal monitoring: A Canadian survey. *CMAJ, 148,* 1737-1742.

Flamm, B.L. (1994). Electronic fetal monitoring in the United States. *Birth, 21,* 105-106.

Hodnett, E.D. (1997). Support from caregivers during childbirth (Cochrane Review). *Cochrane Library,* Issue 3, 1998. Oxford: Update Software.

National Institute of Child Health and Human Development Research Planning Workshop. (1997). Electronic fetal heart rate monitoring: Research guidelines for interpretation. *Journal of Obstetric, Gynecologic, and Neonatal Nursing, 26,* 635-640 and *American Journal of Obstetrics and Gynecology, 177,* 1385-1390.

Society of Obstetricians and Gynaecologists of Canada. (1995). Fetal health surveillance in labor. (SOGC Policy Statement). *Journal SOGC, 17,* 865-901.

Thacker, S.B., & Stroup, D.F. (1998). Continuous electronic fetal heart monitoring during labor (Cochrane Review). *Cochrane Library,* Issue 3, 1998. Oxford: Update Software.

Resources

For more information about AWHONN programs and resources regarding fetal heart monitoring, call AWHONN headquarters at 1-800-673-8499 (US) or 1-800-245-0231 (Canada). To obtain information on current ACOG resources addressing fetal monitoring, contact the ACOG Resource Center at 1-202-863-2518. For information on SOGC resources, call 1-800-561-2416.

Appendix H

Selected Pattern Interpretation at 1 Centimeter per Minute Paper Speed

Cardiotocography (electronic fetal heart rate [FHR] monitoring) outside of North America is usually done at a paper speed of 1 cm/min, which is different from the 3 cm/min paper speed used in North America. Note that the FHR range is from 50 to 210 bpm and that each vertical line on the trace paper is 30 seconds of time. Terms used in this section:

Toco transducer—tocograph transducer (same as tocodynamometer)

IUPT—intrauterine pressure transducer (same as IUPC)

Reactive Fetal Heart Rate on Admission

SIGNAL SOURCE	Spiral electrode and tocotransducer
FHR	Baseline: 120 to 130 bpm
	Variability: Moderate
	Nonperiodic changes: Acceleration of FHR with uterine contractions and fetal movement
UTERINE ACTIVITY	Frequency: 3½ to 4 minutes
	Duration: 60 to 90 seconds

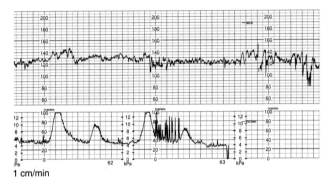

1 cm/min

Figure H-1
(Courtesy Dr. Lennart Nordström, Stockholm, Sweden.)

Reactive Non-Stress Test

SIGNAL SOURCE   Ultrasound and tocotransducer

FHR   Baseline: 135 to 140 bpm

    Variability: Moderate

    Nonperiodic changes: Accelerations of FHR

Baseline rate shows a quiet period without accelerations and baseline variability of 5 to 10 bpm followed by an active period indicated by Fetal Movement Profile (FMP) blocks. Note that there are more than two accelerations of >15 bpm lasting >15 seconds and an increase of variability.

UTERINE ACTIVITY   Not in active labor

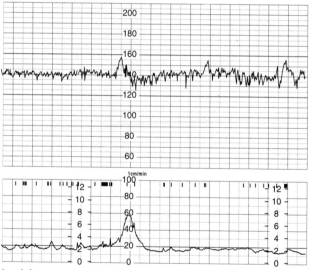

1 cm/min

Figure H-2
(Courtesy Agilent Technologies, Böblingen, Germany.)

Normal Fetal Heart Rate Tracing

SIGNAL SOURCE	Spiral electrode and IUPT
FHR	Baseline: 132 bpm
	Variability: Moderate
	Nonperiodic changes: Accelerations of FHR
UTERINE ACTIVITY	Frequency: 2 to 3 minutes
	Duration: 60 seconds
	Intensity: 58 mm Hg
	Resting tone: 15 mm Hg

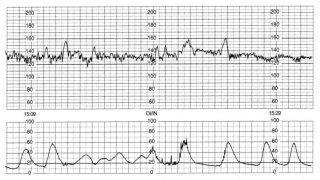

1 cm/min

Figure H-3
(Courtesy Dr. Herman P. van Geijn, Amsterdam, The Netherlands.)

Normal Trace of First Stage of Labor

SIGNAL SOURCE   Ultrasound and tocotransducer

FHR   Baseline: 100 to 110 bpm

        Variability: Moderate

        Nonperiodic changes: Acceleration of FHR
        with fetal movement

UTERINE ACTIVITY   Frequency: 3 to 4 minutes

        Duration: 60 seconds

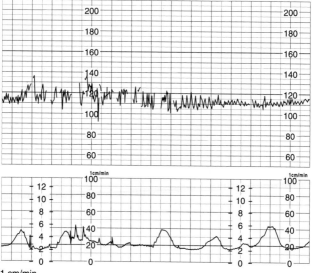

1 cm/min

Figure H-4

(Courtesy Agilent Technologies, Böblingen, Germany.)

Uterine Hypertonia

SIGNAL SOURCE	Spiral electrode and IUPT
FHR	Baseline: 130 bpm
	Variability: Moderate
	Periodic changes: None
UTERINE ACTIVITY	Frequency: 1 to 2 minutes
	Duration: 60 seconds
	Intensity: 50 to 60 mm Hg
	Resting tone: 5 to 10 mm Hg
	Note increase in resting tone with clustering of frequent uterine contractions

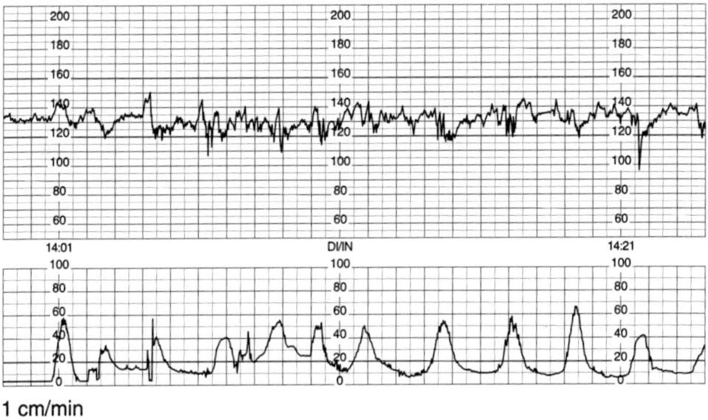

1 cm/min

Figure H-5
(Courtesy Dr. Herman P. van Geijn, Amsterdam, The Netherlands.)

Fluctuating Baseline/Variable Decelerations

SIGNAL SOURCE	Spiral electrode and tocotransducer
FHR	Baseline: Fluctuating
	Variability: Moderate
	Nonperiodic changes: Variable decelerations
UTERINE ACTIVITY	Frequency: 3 to 3½ min
	Duration: 60 to 90 seconds

This patient was a primagravida at 9 cm with a prolonged second stage. Fetal blood sampling revealed a pH of 7.25 and lactate of 2.8 milliosmols/L (within normal limits).

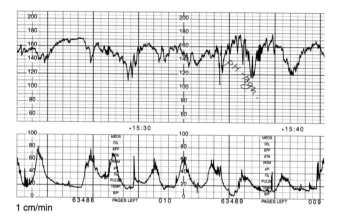

1 cm/min

Figure H-6
(Courtesy Dr. Lennart Nordström, Stockholm, Sweden.)

Sinusoidal Pattern

SIGNAL SOURCE   Ultrasound and tocotransducer

FHR   Baseline: 180 bpm—tachycardia

                       Variability: Sinusoidal pattern

                       Periodic changes: None

                       Fetus had severe anemia

UTERINE ACTIVITY   Not in active labor; note the characteristic
                       zig-zag maternal respiratory movements
                       on the uterine activity tracing

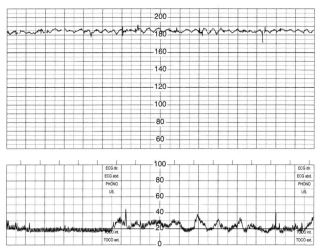

1 cm/min

Figure H-7
(Courtesy Agilent Technologies, Böblingen, Germany.)

Tachycardia

SIGNAL SOURCE   Spiral electrode and IUPT

FHR   Baseline: 165 bpm

                          Variability: Moderate

                          Nonperiodic changes: Accelerations and
                          mild variable decelerations

UTERINE ACTIVITY   Frequency: 1½ to 2 minutes

                          Duration: 60 seconds

                          Intensity: Unable to determine exactly;
                          approximately 40 to 50 mm Hg

                          Resting Tone: Unable to determine
                          exactly; approximately 5 to 10 mm Hg

                          It does not appear that the UA was zeroed
                          before use

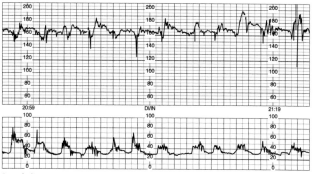

1 cm/min

Figure H-8
(Courtesy Dr. Herman P. van Geijn, Amsterdam, The
Netherlands.)

Early Decelerations

SIGNAL SOURCE   Spiral electrode and tocotransducer

FHR   Baseline: 120 bpm

                       Variability: Moderate

                       Periodic changes: Early decelerations

UTERINE ACTIVITY   Frequency: 4 to 5 minutes

                       Duration: 90 seconds

                       Note the mirror image of the early decel-
                            erations with the uterine contractions

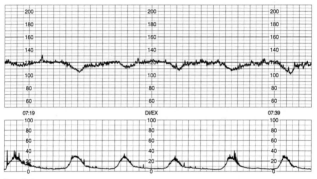

1 cm/min

Figure H-9
(Courtesy Dr. Herman P. van Geijn, Amsterdam, The
Netherlands.)

Late Decelerations

SIGNAL SOURCE   Spiral electrode and IUPT

FHR   Baseline: 165 bpm

    Variability: Moderate

    Periodic changes: Repetitive late decelerations

    Note that the nadir of the deceleration "mirrors" the amplitude of the uterine contraction

UTERINE ACTIVITY   Frequency: 2 to 4 minutes

    Duration: 45 to 60 seconds

    Intensity: 70 mm Hg

    Resting tone: 15 mm Hg

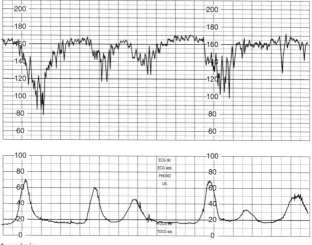

1 cm/min

Figure H-10
(Courtesy Agilent Technologies, Böblingen, Germany.)

Mild Variable Decelerations

SIGNAL SOURCE	Spiral electrode and IUPT
FHR	Baseline: 135 to 140 bpm
	Variability: Moderate
	Nonperiodic changes: Mild variable decelerations with shouldering and overshoot
UTERINE ACTIVITY	Frequency: 2 minutes
	Duration: 45 to 60 seconds
	Intensity: 80 mm Hg
	Resting tone: 5 to 10 mm Hg

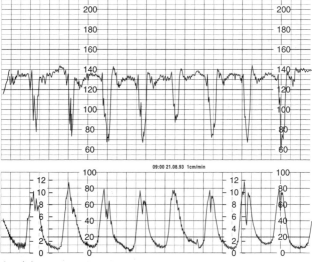

Figure H-11
(Courtesy Agilent Technologies, Böblingen, Germany.)

Variable Decelerations

SIGNAL SOURCE   Spiral electrode and IUPT

FHR   Baseline: 140 to 150 bpm

      Variability: Moderate

      Nonperiodic changes: Mild to moderate variable decelerations; note shouldering

UTERINE ACTIVITY   Frequency: 2 to 3 minutes

      Duration: 60 to 90 seconds

      Intensity: 60 to 80 mm Hg

      Resting tone: 15 to 20 mm Hg

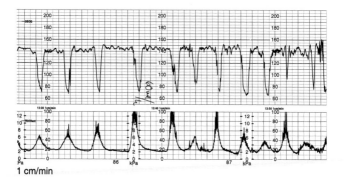

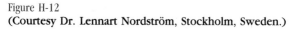

1 cm/min

Figure H-12
(Courtesy Dr. Lennart Nordström, Stockholm, Sweden.)

Variable Decelerations

SIGNAL SOURCE   Spiral electrode and tocotransducer

FHR   Baseline: 140 to 150 bpm

                     Variability: Moderate

                     Nonperiodic changes: Variable decelerations with shouldering

UTERINE ACTIVITY   Frequency: 2 to 3½ minutes

                     Duration: 60 to 90 seconds

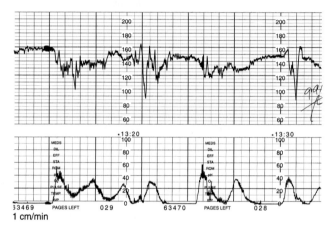

Figure H-13

(Courtesy Dr. Lennart Nordström, Stockholm, Sweden.)

Moderate/Severe Variable Decelerations

SIGNAL SOURCE	Spiral electrode and tocotransducer
FHR	Baseline: 160 bpm (it was 140 bpm earlier in labor) progressing to unstable baseline FHR
	Variability: Moderate with episode of decreasing variability, slow return to baseline, and overshoot with some decelerations
	Nonperiodic changes: Moderate to severe variable decelerations; note the shapes of the decelerations in U, V, and W shapes characteristic of variable decelerations. Most of the decelerations last 60 seconds except the W-shaped decelerations that last appreciably longer.
UTERINE ACTIVITY	Frequency: 2 to 4 minutes
	Duration: about 60 to 90 seconds
	It is difficult to assess uterine activity in the first panel; this may be due to location of the tocotransducer and patient movement

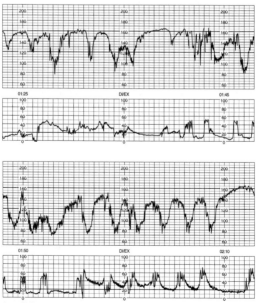

1 cm/min

Amnioinfusion for Variable Decelerations

SIGNAL SOURCE   Spiral electrode and IUPT

FHR   Baseline: Unstable initially, changing to
                     120 bpm after amnioinfusion

                     Variability: Moderate to marked (saltatory)

                     Nonperiodic changes: Variable decelera-
                     tions

                     Note the progression to a severe variable
                     deceleration that was immediately re-
                     lieved by the amnioinfusion bolus of
                     500 ml of fluid

UTERINE ACTIVITY   Frequency: 2 to 3 minutes

                     Duration: 60 to 90 seconds

                     Intensity: 60 mm Hg

                     Resting tone: 20 mm Hg

                     It does not appear that the UA baseline
                     was zeroed before implementation of
                     cardiotography

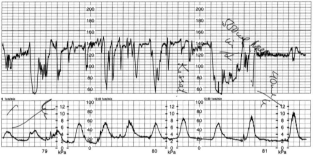

1 cm/min

Figure H-15
(Courtesy Dr. Lennart Nordström, Stockholm, Sweden.)

Figure H-14, p. 326
(Courtesy Dr. Herman P. van Geijn, Amsterdam, The
Netherlands.)

Prolonged Deceleration Secondary to Uterine Hyperstimulation

SIGNAL SOURCE	Spiral electrode and IUPT
FHR	Baseline: 140 bpm
	Variability: Moderate to marked
	Nonperiodic changes: Prolonged deceleration below normal FHR range for 5 minutes
UTERINE ACTIVITY	Frequency: 1½ to 2 minutes
	Duration: 60 to 90 seconds
	Intensity: 70 mm Hg
	Resting tone: 20 mm Hg increasing to 40 mm Hg before intervention

Oxytocin was discontinued immediately when hypertonus was observed but without effect on UA and FHR. A bolus of terbutaline 0.25 mg in 5 ml IV (indicated by the arrow) relaxed the uterus within 2 minutes, and the FHR pattern returned to normal.

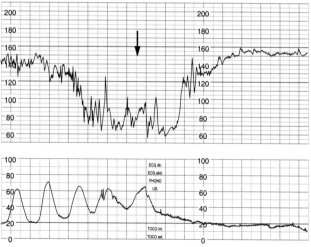

1 cm/min

Figure H-16

(Courtesy Agilent Technologies, Böblingen, Germany.)

Glossary of Terms and Abbreviations

abruptio placentae premature separation of the placenta before delivery of the fetus

acceleration transient increase in the fetal heart rate (FHR)

acidemia increased concentration of hydrogen ions in the blood

acidosis a pathological condition marked by an increased concentration of hydrogen ions in tissue

ADT admission, discharge, transfer

AFI amniotic fluid index

amniocentesis procedure in which amniotic fluid is removed from the uterine cavity by insertion of a needle through the abdominal and uterine walls into the amniotic sac

amnioinfusion replacement of amniotic fluid with normal saline through an intrauterine pressure catheter

amnion inner of the two fetal membranes forming the sac that encloses the fetus within the uterus

amniotomy artificial rupture of the amniotic sac

anencephaly absence of the cerebrum, cerebellum, and flat bones of the skull

angiography x-ray examination of blood vessels made radiopaque by the injection of a radiopaque substance

ANS autonomic nervous system

antepartum occurring before birth

Apgar score quantitative estimate of the condition of an infant at 1 and 5 minutes after birth, derived by assigning points to the quality of heart rate, respiratory effort, color, muscle tone, and response to stimulation; expressed as the sum of these points with the maximum, or best, score being 10

AROM artificial rupture of membranes

artifact irregularities on a fetal monitor tracing caused by electrical interference or poor reception of the FHR signal; may appear as scattered dots or lines

ASAP as soon as possible

asphyxia   condition in which there is hypoxia and metabolic acidosis

AST   acoustic stimulation test; same as vibroacoustic stimulation test

AV   atrioventricular

atelectasis   collapse of the alveoli, or air sacs, of the lungs

augmentation   correcting of ineffective uterine contractions (caused by dystocia) that occur after the start of spontaneous labor (ACOG, 1995a)

baroceptor   a pressure receptor; a nerve ending located in the walls of the carotid sinus and the aortic arch that is sensitive to stretching induced by changes in blood pressure

baseline FHR   range of FHR present between periodic changes over a 10-minute period

bilirubin   pigment produced by the breakdown of hemoglobin in cell elements and in red blood cells

biparietal diameter   distance from one parietal eminence to another; can be measured by ultrasound to determine gestational age

BL   baseline (baseline FHR)

BP   blood pressure

BPP   biophysical profile

bpm   beats per minute

bradycardia   baseline FHR below 120 bpm for 10 minutes

cardiotography   another term for electronic FHR monitoring

CBC   complete blood count

CC   cord compression

C/C/+1   used to indicate results of vaginal examination (e.g., cervix completely effaced/completely dilated/+1 station)

cephalopelvic disproportion (CPD)   disparity between the size of the fetal head and the maternal pelvis, preventing vaginal delivery

cervical ripening   a complex process that culminates in the physical softening and distensibility of the cervix

chain-of-command   a reporting mechanism to resolve conflicts

chemoceptor   sensory end organ capable of reacting to a chemical stimulus

chorion   outer of the two membranes forming the sac that encloses the fetus within the uterus

chromosome a dark-stained body within the cell nucleus that carries hereditary factors (genes); there are 46 chromosomes in each cell except in the mature ovum and sperm, where that number is halved

circumvallate placenta placenta in which an overgrowth of the decidua separates the placental margin from the chorionic plate, producing a thick, white ring around the circumference of the placenta and a reduction in distribution of fetal blood vessels to the placental periphery

cm centimeter

CMV cytomegalovirus

CNS central nervous system

coupling two uterine contractions, one right after the other; the interval of time between the coupled contractions is less than the interval to the next uterine contraction or next set of coupled contractions

CP cerebral palsy

CRP C-reactive protein

CST contraction stress test

CT computed tomography

CTG cardiotocography; another term for electronic FHR monitoring

CVS chorionic villus sampling

d/c or D/C discontinue(d)

deceleration a drop in the FHR; usually occurs in response to a uterine contraction

DFMC daily fetal movement count

DIL cervical dilatation

Doppler ultrasound type of ultrasound that is reflected from moving interfaces such as closure of fetal heart valves; Doppler ultrasound is used in electronic FHR monitors

DR delivery room

DTR deep tendon reflex

DW dextrose in water

ECG electrocardiogram

ED early deceleration

EDC expected date of confinement

EFF effacement of the cervix

effleurage gentle stroking of the abdomen; used during labor in the Lamaze method of prepared childbirth

EFM electronic fetal monitor(ing)

epidural   area situated on or over the dura mater; regional anesthetic is often injected into the peridural (epidural) space of the spinal cord

episodic changes   spontaneous (nonperiodic) changes in the FHR that occur at any time; they are not related to uterine contractions, e.g., accelerations and variable decelerations

FAST   Fetal Acoustic Stimulation Test

FBM   fetal breathing movements

FECG   fetal electrocardiogram

FHR   fetal heart rate

FHT   fetal heart tones

FM   fetal movement

FMP   fetal movement profile

frequency (of contractions)   time from the onset of one uterine contraction to the onset of the next

FSpO$_2$ fetal oxygen saturation

FT   fetal tone

GBS   group B streptococcus

gestation   pregnancy; the period of intrauterine fetal development from conception to birth

gestational age   age of a conceptus computed from the first day of the last menstrual period to any point in time thereafter

gtt   drops

HC   head compression

HR   heart rate

HUAM   home uterine activity monitoring

hydramnios   excessive volume of amniotic fluid, usually greater than 1.2 L; it is frequently seen in diabetic pregnancies and in fetuses with open neural tube defects

hydrocephaly   increased accumulation of cerebrospinal fluid within the ventricles of the brain; may result from congenital anomalies, infection, injury, or brain tumor; the head is usually large and globular with a disproportionately small face; the increased head diameter is possible in the fetus and infant because the sutures of the skull have not closed

hydrostatic pressure   pressure created in a fluid system

hyperthermia   hyperpyrexia; high fever

hypertonic   solution with a high osmotic pressure

hypertonus   excessive muscular tonus or tension

hypothermia   subnormal temperature of the body

hypotonic   solution with a low osmotic pressure

hypoxemia   decreased oxygen content in the blood

hypoxia   a pathological condition marked by a decreased level of oxygen in tissue

IM   intramuscular

induction   consists of stimulation of uterine contractions before the spontaneous onset of labor for the purpose of accomplishing delivery (ACOG, 1995b)

intervillous space   space between the myometrium and placental villi that is filled with maternal blood

intrapartum   occurring during labor or delivery

IUGR   intrauterine growth restriction

IUP   intrauterine pressure

IUPC   intrauterine pressure catheter

IUPT   intrauterine pressure transducer

IV   intravenous (parenteral fluids)

IVP   intravenous pyelogram

L   liter

LATS   long-acting thyroid-stimulating hormone

LD   late deceleration

LDR   labor/delivery/recovery room

L/S   lecithin/sphingomyelin ratio

LTV   long-term variability

macrosomia   large body size as seen in some postmature infants and in those born to diabetic mothers

MECG   maternal electrocardiogram

meconium   pasty greenish mass that collects in the fetal intestine, usually expelled during the first 3 to 4 days after birth; its presence in amniotic fluid is abnormal and is usually considered a sign of fetal distress

meningomyelocele   protrusion of a portion of the spinal cord and membranes through a defect in the vertebral column

MHR   maternal heart rate

min   minutes

mm Hg   millimeters of mercury (unit of measure of pressure)

morbidity   state of being diseased or sick; the number of sick persons or cases of disease in relationship to a specific population

mortality   the death rate; the ratio of number of deaths to a given population

MRI   magnetic resonance imaging

MSpO$_2$ maternal pulse oximetry

mU   milliunits (unit of oxytocin dosage)

MVU   Montevideo units

nadir   the lowest point of a curve; the depth or trough of a FHR deceleration

NBP   maternal noninvasive blood pressure

nonperiodic   episodic or spontaneous changes in FHR that are not associated with uterine contractions, such as accelerations and variable decelerations

NRP   Neonatal Resucitation Program

NS   normal saline

NST   Non-Stress test

nuchal   neck (as in umbilical cord around the fetal neck)

OCT   oxytocin challenge test

OD   optical density

osmolality   quantity of a solute existing in solution as molecules or ions or both; the concentration of a solution

osmotic pressure   pressure developed when two solutions of different concentrations of the same solute are separated by a membrane permeable to the solvent only

overshoot   transient acceleratory phase of the FHR that occurs at the end of some variable decelerations

P   pulse

PAC   premature atrial contraction

PAT   paroxysmal atrial tachycardia

PCB   paracervical block anesthesia

PDA   patent ductus arteriosus

PE   pelvic examination

peak   the highest point of a uterine contraction or FHR acceleration

periodic changes   changes in the FHR that are associated with uterine contractions such as early and late decelerations

PG   phosphatidyl glycerol

PI   phosphatidyl inositol

piezoelectric   a substance that has the ability to convert energy from one form into another, such as mechanical pressure into electrical energy and vice versa, as with the ultrasound transducer

PIH   pregnancy-induced hypertension

Pit   Pitocin (oxytocin)

PL   disaturated (acetone precipitated) lecithin

placenta previa   placenta covering the internal cervical os

PMI   point of maximal intensity

PO   by mouth

polyhydramnios   *see* **hydramnios**

prn   as necessary

PROM   premature rupture of membranes

PTL   preterm labor

PVC   premature ventricular contraction

q   every

R   respirations

RDS   respiratory distress syndrome

reactivity   fetus demonstrates episodes of FHR acceleration associated with fetal movement or stimuli; reactivity is associated with fetal well-being and forms the basis for the NST and VAS

resting tone   intrauterine pressure between contractions (tonus)

R/O   rule out, consider as a possibility

ROM   rupture of membranes

SA   sinoatrial

saltatory   sudden abrupt changes in baseline FHR with marked, exaggerated, or excessive variability greater than 25 beats/minute

sawtooth   a FHR pattern that resembles the teeth on a saw and is generally associated with arrhythmias

SE   spiral electrode or scalp electrode

sec   seconds

SGA   small for gestational age

shouldering   transient preacceleratory and postacceleratory phase of FHR at the beginning and end of some variable decelerations

sinusoidal HR pattern   baseline FHR that has a predominance of long-term variability with a characteristic sine wave pattern

spina bifida   congenital defect in the closure of the vertebral canal with a herniated protrusion of the meninges of the cord

spinal anesthesia   anesthesia produced by the injection of an anesthetic into the spinal subarachnoid space

SQ   subcutaneous

SROM   spontaneous rupture of membranes

STA   station

STV   short-term variability

supine hypotension   weight and pressure of uterus on the ascending vena cava when the patient is in a supine position decreases venous return, cardiac output, and blood pressure

surfactant phospholipid that normally lines the alveolar sacs after 34 weeks' gestation. Its presence prevents collapse (atelectasis) of the alveoli by permitting a small amount of air to remain in the alveoli on exhalation. The L/S ratio as measured in amniotic fluid tests for the presence of surfactant. Neonates born without surfactant develop respiratory distress syndrome (RDS)

SVT supraventricular tachycardia

T temperature

tachycardia baseline FHR above 160 bpm for 10 minutes

tachysystole excessive uterine contraction frequency; six or more uterine contractions in consecutive 10-minute intervals

tetany state of increased neuromuscular irritability or spasm

toco tocotransducer or tocodynamometer, external device used to record uterine activity

tocodynamometer pressure-sensing instrument for measuring the duration and frequency of uterine contractions

tocolytics drugs used to inhibit uterine contractions and stop labor

tocotransducer *see* **tocodynamometer**

tonus intrauterine pressure between contractions (resting tone)

transducer device that converts energy from one form to another; sound or pressure can be converted into an electrical impulse and vice versa

trough lowest point of a deceleration

UA uterine activity

UC uterine contraction

ultrasound transducer instrument that uses high-frequency sound (ultrasound) to detect moving interfaces, such as the closure of fetal heart valves, to monitor the FHR

UPI uteroplacental insufficiency

US ultrasound

UTI urinary tract infection

variability fluctuations in the baseline FHR

VAS vibroacoustic stimulation

VBAC vaginal birth after cesarean

VD variable deceleration

VDRL Venereal Disease Research Laboratories

VE vaginal examination

References and Bibliography

References

Adair DC et al: Oral or vaginal misoprostol administration for induction of labor: a randomized, double-blind trial, *Obstet Gynecol* 92(5):810-813, 1998.

American Academy of Pediatrics, American College of Obstetricians and Gynecologists: *Guidelines for perinatal care,* Washington, DC, 1997, The Academy and The College.

American College of Obstetricians and Gynecologists: *Ultrasonography in pregnancy,* tech bull 187, Washington DC, Dec 1993, The College.

American College of Obstetricians and Gynecologists: *Dystocia and the augmentation of labor,* tech bull 218, Washington DC, Dec 1995a, The College.

American College of Obstetricians and Gynecologists: *Induction of labor,* tech bull 217, Washington DC, Dec 1995b, The College.

American College of Obstetricians and Gynecologists: *Umbilical artery blood acid-base analysis,* tech bull 216, Washington DC, Nov 1995c, The College.

American College of Obstetricians and Gynecologists: *Fetal heart rate patterns: monitoring, interpretation, and management,* tech bulletin 207, Washington DC, July 1995d, The College.

American College of Obstetricians and Gynecologists: *Preterm labor,* tech bull 206, Washington DC, June 1995e, The College.

American College of Obstetricians and Gynecologists: *Assessment of fetal lung maturity,* education bull 230, Washington DC, Nov 1996, The College.

American College of Obstetricians and Gynecologists: *Inappropriate use of the terms fetal distress and birth asphyxia,* Committee Opinion no 197, Washington DC, Feb 1998a, The College.

American College of Obstetricians and Gynecologists: *Tocolysis,* Criteria Set no 31, Washington DC, Feb 1998b, The College.

American College of Obstetricians and Gynecologists: *Induction of labor with misoprostol,* Committee Opinion no 228, Washington, DC, Nov 1999a, The College.

American College of Obstetricians and Gynecologists: *Induction of labor,* Practice Bull No 10, Washington, DC, Nov 1999b, The College.

American College of Obstetricians and Gynecologists: *Antepartum fetal surveillance,* Clinical Management Guideline No 9, Washington, DC, Oct 1999c, The College.

American Institute of Ultrasound in Medicine: *Bioeffects and safety of diagnostic ultrasound,* ed 2, Laurel, Md, 1998, The Institute.

Arias F: Intrauterine resuscitation with terbutaline: a method for the management of acute intrapartum fetal distress, *Am J Obstet Gynecol* 131(1):39-43, 1978.

Association of Women's Health, Obstetric and Neonatal Nurses: *Fetal heart monitoring principles and practices,* ed 2, Dubuque, Iowa, 1997, Kendall/Hunt.

Association of Women's Health, Obstetric and Neonatal Nurses: *Clinical competencies and education guide: fetal surveillance in antepartum and intrapartum nursing practice,* ed 3, Washington DC, 1998, The Association.

Bald R et al: Antepartum fetal blood sampling with cordocentesis: comparison with chorionic villus sampling and amniocentesis in diagnosing karyotype anomalies, *J Reprod Med* 36(9):655-658, 1991.

Benett KA et al: A masked randomized comparison of oral and vaginal administration of misoprostol for labor induction, *Obstet Gynecol* 92(4):481-486, 1998.

Benn PA et al: Prenatal diagnosis of diverse chromosome abnormalities in a population of patients identified by triple-marker testing as screen positive for Down syndrome, *Am J Obstet Gynecol* 173(2):496-501, 1995.

Berkus MD et al: Electronic fetal monitoring: what's reassuring? *Acta Obstet Gynecol Scand* 78(1):15-21, 1999.

Berkus MD et al: Meconium-stained amniotic fluid: increased risk for adverse neonatal outcome, *Obstet Gynecol* 84(1):115-120, 1994.

Besinger RE, Johnson TRB: Doppler recordings of fetal movement: clinical correlation with real-time ultrasound, *Obstet Gynecol* 74(2):277-280, 1989.

Bevis DCA: The antenatal prediction of haemolytic disease of the newborn, *Lancet* 1:395-398, 1952.

Black RS, Lees C, Thompson C, Pickles A, and Campbell S: Maternal and fetal cardiovascular effects of transdermal glyceryl trinitrate and intravenous ritodrine, *Obstet Gynecol* 94(4):572-576, 1999

Bornstein MD, Shuwager MD: Protocol: Misoprostol (Cytotec for Cervical Ripening and Induction of Labor, *www.obgyn.net*/english/ob/misoprostol/ protocol.htm, accessed 3/30/99.

Brown CE: Intrapartal tocolysis: an option for acute intrapartal fetal crisis, *JOGNN* 27(3):257-261, 1998.

Brown HL et al: A randomized comparison of home uterine activity monitoring in the outpatient management of women treated for preterm labor, *Am J Obstet Gynecol* 180(4):798-805, 1999.

Burke M et al: Intrauterine resuscitation with tocolysis: an alternate month clinical trial, *J Perinatal* 9(3):296-300, 1989.

Caldeyro-Barcia R, Poseiro JJ: Physiology of the uterine contraction, *Clin Obstet Gynecol* 3:386-408, 1960.

Cedars-Sinai Medical Center v. Superior Court, *96 Journal DAR,* 1996, p 2949.

Centers for Disease Control and Prevention (CDC): *Infant mortality,* National Vital Statistics Reports 47(23)1-24, 1999.

Centers for Disease Control and Prevention (CDC): *Birth statistics for the nation,* National Vital Statistics Reports 46(suppl 11):100, 1996.

Chez BF: *EFM terminology: communicating if you are reassured or not,* Proceedings of the third annual National Conference of Electronic Fetal Monitoring: the science, the art, the future, Oct 1992, Washington, DC.

Clements JA, Platzker ACG, Tierney DF: Assessment of the risk of the respiratory distress syndrome by a rapid test for surfactant in amniotic fluid, *N Engl J Med* 286:1077, 1972.

Collaborative Home Uterine Monitoring Study (CHUMS) Group: A multicenter randomized controlled trial of home uterine monitoring: active versus sham device, *Am J Obstet Gynecol* 173(4):1120-1127, 1995.

Creasy, RK and Iams JD: Preterm labor and delivery. In Creasy RK and Resnik R editors: *Maternal-Fetal Medicine* (ed 4), Philadelphia, 1999, WB Saunders.

Dickason E, Silverman B, Kaplan J: *Maternal-infant nursing care,* ed 3, St Louis, 1998, Mosby.

Dicker D et al: Effect of intracranial pressure changes on the fetal heart rate: study of a hydrocephalic fetus, *Israel J Med Sci* 19(4):364, 1983.

Didolkar S, Mutch M: Major/multiple congenital anomalies and intrapartum fetal heart rate patterns, *South Dakota J Med* 33(9):5-9, 1979.

Dildy GA, Clark SL, Loucks CA: Intrapartum fetal pulse oximetry: past, present, and future, *Am J Obstet Gynecol* 175(1):1-9, 1996.

Dildy GA et al: Current status of the multicenter randomized clinical trial on fetal oxygen saturation monitoring in the United States, *Eur J Obstet Gynecol Reprod Biol* 72(suppl 1):S43-S50, 1997.

Dildy GA et al: A multicenter randomized trial of fetal pulse oximetry, *Am J Obstet Gynecol* 182(1):S1, 2000.

Dyson DC et al: Prevention of preterm birth in high risk patients: the role of education and provider contact versus home uterine monitoring, *Am J Obstet Gynecol* 164(3):756-762, 1991.

Dyson DC et al: Monitoring women at risk for preterm labor, *N Engl J Med* 338(1):15-19, 1998.

ECRI (Emergency Care Research Institute): *Fetal monitoring: hospital risk control.* Philadelphia, 1995, Pennsylvania Insurance Management Co.

Freeman RK, Garite TJ, Nageotte MP: *Fetal heart rate monitoring,* Baltimore, 1991, Williams and Wilkins.

Fresquez M: *OB/GYN limited ultrasound series,* Washington DC, 1996, Association of Obstetric, Gynecologic and Neonatal Nurses.

Garite T, Ray D: Intrauterine resuscitation with tocolytics, *Contemporary OB/GYN* 71:24-28, 1988.

Gegor CL, Paine LL: Antepartum fetal testing techniques: an update for today's perinatal nurse, *J Perinat Neonat Nurs* 5(4):1-15, 1992.

Giger JN, Davidhizer RE: *Transcultural nursing,* ed 3, St Louis, 1999, Mosby.

Gilstrap LC et al: Diagnosis of birth asphyxia on the basis of fetal pH, Apgar score, and newborn cerebral dysfunction, *Am J Obstet Gynecol* 161(3):825, 1989.

Gluck L et al: Diagnosis of respiratory distress syndrome by amniocentesis, *Am J Obstet Gyneol* 109(3):441, 1971.

Goff v Doctors' Hospital, 166 Cal App 314, 333, P2d, 1958.

Goldenberg RL et al: The preterm prediction study: fetal fibronectin testing and spontaneous preterm birth, *Obstet Gynecol* 87(5):643-648, 1996.

Hankins GDV: Apgar scores: are they enough? *Contemp Ob/Gyn: Ob-Gyn Law Special Issue* 36:13-25, 1991.

Harvey C, Chez BF: *Critical concepts in fetal heart rate monitoring,* Washington, DC, 1997, Association of Women's Health, Obstetric and Neonatal Nurses.

Helwig IT et al: Umbilical cord blood acid base state: what is normal? *Am J Obstet Gynecol* 174(6):1807-1814, 1996.

Huddleston JF: Contraction stress test by intermittent nipple stimulation, *Obstet Gynecol* 63(5):669-673, 1984.

Iams JD, Johnson FF, O'Shaugnessy RW: A prospective random trial of home uterine activity monitoring in pregnancies at increased risk of preterm labor, *Am J Obstet Gynecol* 159(3):595-603, 1988.

Irion O, Pedrazzoli J, Mermillod B: A randomized trial comparing vaginal and cervical prostaglandin gel for cervical ripening and labor induction, *Obstet Gynecol* 91(1):65-71, 1998.

Kelly CS: Perinatal computerized patient record and archiving systems: pitfalls and enhancements for implementing a successful computerized medical record, *J Perinat Neonat Nurs* 12(4):1-14, 1999.

Kleinman CS, Nehgme R, Copel JA: Fetal cardiac arrhythmias: diagnosis and therapy. In Creasy RK, Resnik R, eds: *Maternal-fetal medicine,* ed 4, Philadelphia, 1999, WB Saunders.

Kruger K, Kublickas M, Westgren M: Lactate in scalp and cord blood from fetuses with ominous fetal heart rate patterns, *Obstet Gynecol* 92(6):912-922, 1998.

Kubli FW et al: Observations on heart rate and pH in the human fetus during labor, *Am J Obstet Gynecol* 104(8):1190-1206, 1969.

Kühnert M, Seelback-Goebel BS, Butterwegge M: Predictive agreement between the fetal arterial oxygen saturation and fetal scalp pH: results of the German multicenter study, *Am J Obstet Gynecol* 178(2):330-335, 1998a.

Kühnert M et al: Guidelines for the use of fetal pulse oximetry during labor and delivery, *Prenat Neonat Med* 3(4):432-433, 1998b.

Lowdermilk D, Perry S, Bobak I: *Maternity nursing,* ed 5, St Louis, 1999, Mosby.

Lowdermilk D, Perry S, Bobak I: *Maternity and women's health care,* ed 7, St Louis, 2000, Mosby.

Lurie S, Rabinerson D: Balloon ripening of the cervix (letter), *Lancet* 349(9050):509, 1997.

MacDonald D: Cerebral palsy and intrapartum fetal monitoring, *N Engl J Med* 334(10):659-660, 1996.

McNamara H, Johnson N, Lilford R: The effect on fetal arteriolar oxygen saturation resulting from giving oxygen to the mother measured by pulse oximetry, *Br J Obstet Gynaecol* 100(5):446-449, 1993.

Melendez TD, Rayburn WF, Smith CV: Characterization of fetal body movement recorded by the Hewlett-Packard M-11350-A fetal monitor, *Am J Obstet Gynecol* 167(3):700-702, 1992.

Miyasaki FS, Nevarez F: Saline amnioinfusion for relief of repetitive variable decelerations: a prospective randomized study, *Am J Obstet Gynecol* 153(3):301-306, 1985.

Miyasaki FS, Taylor NA: Saline amnioinfusion for relief of variable or prolonged decelerations, *Am J Obstet Gynecol* 146(6):670-678, 1983.

Mooney RA et al: Effectiveness of combining maternal serum alpha-fetoprotein and hCG in a second-trimester screening program for Down syndrome, *Obstet Gynecol* 83(6):298, 1994.

Moore ML: Biochemical markers for preterm labor and birth: what is their role in the care of pregnant women? *Am J Matern Child Nurs* 24(2):80-86, 1999.

Morrison JC et al: Prediction of spontaneous preterm birth by fetal fibronectin and uterine activity, *Obstet Gynecol* 87(5):649-655, 1996.

National Institute of Child Health and Human Development Research Planning Workshop: Electronic fetal heart rate monitoring: research guidelines for interpretation, *Am J Obstet Gynecol* 177(6):1385-1390, 1997.

Nellcor: *Fetal oxygen sensor FS 14 series placement guide,* Pleasanton, Calif, 1998, Nellcor-A Unit of Mallinckrodt, Inc.

Nijuis JG et al: Case reports: a sinusoidal-like fetal heart rate pattern in association with fetal suckling—report of 2 cases, *Eur J Obstet Gynecol Reprod Biol* 16:353-358, 1984.

Niswander KR: EFM and brain damage in term and post-term infants, *Contemp Ob/Gyn: Ob/Gyn Law Special Issue* 36:39-50, 1991.

Ombelet W, VanDer Merwe J: Sinusoidal fetal heart rate pattern associated with congenital hydrocephalus, *S Afr Med J* 67:423, 1985.

Orimi v Mission Viejo Hospital, Orange Country Superior Court, *Professional Liability Newsletter,* March 1985.

Parer JT: *Handbook of fetal heart rate monitoring,* Philadelphia, 1997, WB Saunders.

Peaceman AM: Fetal fibronectin as a predictor of preterm birth in patients

342   References and Bibliography

with symptoms: a multicenter trial, *Am J Obstet Gynecol* 177(1):13-18, 1997.

Porto M et al: The role of home uterine activity monitoring in the prevention of preterm birth, In *Abstracts of the Society of Perinatal Obstetricians,* seventh annual meeting, Feb 5-7, 1987, Lake Buena Vista, Fla.

Rubsamen DS: The obstetrician's professional liability: awareness and prevention, *Professional Liability Newsletter, Inc.,* 1993, Orange County Superior Court, no 30-29-74.

Saling E, Schneider D: Biochemical supervision of the foetus during labour, *J Obstet Gynecol Br Commonwealth* 74:749, 1967.

Sanchez-Ramos L et al: Labor induction with prostaglandin E1 misoprostol compared with dinoprostone vaginal insert: a randomized trial, *Ob Gyn* 91(3):401-405, 1998.

Schifrin BS, Weissman BA, Wiley J: Electronic fetal monitoring and obstetrical malpractice, *Law Med Health Care* 13(3), June 1985.

Shellhass CS, Iams JD: Ambulatory management of preterm labor, *Clin Obstet and Gynecol* 41(3):491-495, 1998.

Simpson KR: Intrapartum fetal oxygen saturation monitoring, *Lifelines* 2(6):21-24, 1998.

Society of Obstetricians & Gynecologists of Canada, SOGC Policy statement: Fetal health surveillance in labour, *J SOGC* 17(9):865-910, 1995.

Stanco LM et al: Does Doppler-detected fetal movement decrease the incidence of nonreactive non-stress test? *Obstet Gynecol* 82(6):999-1103, 1993.

Stringer M et al: Maternal-fetal physical assessment in the home setting: role of the advanced practice nurse, *JOGNN* 23(8):720-725, 1994.

Summers L: Methods of cervical ripening and labor induction, *J Nurse-Midwifery* 42(2):71-85, 1997.

Swedlow DB: Review of evidence for a fetal Sp02 critical threshold of 30%, Pleasanton, Calif, 1998, Nellcor–A Unit of Mallinckrodt, Inc.

Tucker SM et al: *Patient care standards,* St Louis, 2000, Mosby.

Valenzuela GJ, Foster T: Use of magnesium sulfate to treat hyperstimulation in term labor, *Obstet Gynecol* 75(5):762-764, 1990.

VanderMoer P, Gerretsen G, Visser G: Fixed fetal heart rate pattern after intrauterine accidental decerebration, *Obstet Gynecol* 65(1):125, 1985.

van Geijn HP: Cardiotocography. In Kurjak A, ed: *Textbook of perinatal medicine,* London, 1998, Parthenon.

van Woerden EE et al: Fetal heart rhythms during behavioral state, *Eur J Obstet Gynecol Reprod Biol* 28:29-38, 1988.

Vintzileos AM et al: Intrapartum electronic fetal heart rate monitoring versus intermittent auscultation: a meta-analysis, *Obstet Gynecol* 85(1):149-155, 1995.

Wallerstedt C et al: Amnioinfusion: an update, *JOGNN* 23(7):573-577, 1994.

Westgren M, Kublickas M, Kruger K: Role of lactate measurements during labor, *Obstet Gynecol Surv* 54(1)43-48, 1999.

Yoon BH el al: Relationship between the fetal biophysical profile score, umbilical artery Doppler velocimetry and fetal blood acid-base status determined by cordocentesis, *Am J Obstet Gynecol* 169(6):1586-1594, 1993.

Zieman M et al: Absorption kinetics of misoprostol with oral or vaginal administration, *Obstet Gynecol* 90(1):88-92, 1997.

Bibliography

Afriat CI: *Electronic fetal monitoring,* Rockville Md, 1989, Aspen.

American College of Obstetricians and Gynecologists: *Management of herpes in pregnancy,* Clinical Management Guideline no 8, Washington, DC, Oct 1999, The College.

American College of Obstetricians and Gynecologists: *Vaginal birth after previous cesarean delivery,* Clinical Management Guideline no 5, Washington, DC, July 1999, The College.

Association of Women's Health, Obstetric and Neonatal Nurses, Washington DC: Website: www.awhonn.org

Association of Women's Health, Obstetric and Neonatal Nurses: *Standards and guidelines for professional nursing practice in the care of women and newborns,* Washington, DC, 1998, The Association.

Cabaniss ML: *Fetal monitoring interpretation,* Philadelphia, 1993, JB Lippincott.

DeStaffany S: Teaching women on bedrest, *Childbirth Instructor,* Spring 1993, pp 38-41.

Feinstein N, Sprague A, Trepanier MJ: *Fetal auscultation,* Washington, DC, 1999, Association of Women's Health, Obstetric and Neonatal Nurses.

Geissler E: *Pocket guide to cultural assessment,* ed 2, St Louis, 1998, Mosby.

Gibb D, Arulkumaran S: *Fetal monitoring in practice,* Oxford, 1998, Butterworth-Heinemann.

Gilbert ES, Harmon JS: *High risk pregnancy and delivery,* St Louis, 1998, Mosby.

Gyetvai K et al: Tocoytics for preterm labor: a systematic review, *Obstet Gynecol* 94(5):869-877, 1999.

Hon EH: *An introduction to fetal heart rate monitoring,* Wallingford, Conn, 1975, Corometrics Medical Systems.

Iams JD, Johnson FF, Parker M: A prospective evaluation of the signs and symptoms of preterm labor, *Obstet Gynecol* 84(2):227-230, 1994.

Knuppel RA, Drukker JE: *High risk pregnancy: a team approach,* Philadelphia, 1993, WB Saunders.

Mayberry LJ et al: Managing second-stage labor, *Lifelines* 3(6):28-34, 2000.

McRae MJ: Litigation, electronic fetal monitoring, and the obstetrical nurse, *JOGNN* 22(5):410-419, Sept/Oct 1993.

Miller LA: Electronic fetal monitoring competency: to validate or not to validate—the opinions of experts, *J Perinat Neonat Nurs* 8(3):12-15, 1994.

Morales WJ: Preparing the fetus for preterm birth, *Baillieres Clin Obstet Gynecol* 7(3):601-610, 1993.

Murray M: *Antepartal and intrapartal fetal monitoring,* Albuquerque, NM, 1997, Learning Resources International, Inc.

OB/GYN Net: Special report: fetal pulse oximetry, I. Roundtable discussion at nineteenth annual meeting of the Society of Maternal-Fetal Medicine, Jan 1999, San Francisco, *www.obgyn.net* Feb 1999 archives.

OB/GYN Net: Special report: fetal pulse oximetry, II. The European experience, *www.obgyn.net* March 1999 archives.

Payton RG, Brucker MC: Drugs and uterine motility, *J Obstet Gynecol Neonat Nurs* 28(6):628-638, 1999.

Perinatal Advisory Council of Los Angeles Communities, Encino Calif, Website: http://web.webaccess.com/PACLAC

Rabello YA, Lapidus MR: *Fundamentals of electronic fetal monitoring,* Wallingford, Conn, 1991, Corometric Medical Systems.

Rommal C: *Professional liability in perinatal practice,* Washington DC, 1998, Association of Women's Health, Obstetric and Neonatal Nurses.

Rostant DM, Cady, RF: *Liability issues in perinatal nursing,* Washington DC, 1998, Association of Women's Health, Obstetric and Neonatal Nurses.

Sanchez-Ramos L et al: Cervical ripening and labor induction with a controlled release dinoprostone vaginal insert: a meta-analysis, *Obstet Gynecol* 5(2)878-883, 1999.

Schifrin BS: *Exercises in fetal monitoring,* St Louis, 1990, Mosby.

Schifrin BS: *More exercises in fetal monitoring,* St Louis, 1993, Mosby.

Simpson KR, Creehan P: *Perinatal nursing,* Washington, DC, 1996, Association of Women's Health, Obstetric and Neonatal Nurses.

Simpson KR, Creehan P: *Competence validation for perinatal care providers: orientation, continuing education and evaluation,* Washington, DC, 1998, Association of Women's Health, Obstetric and Neonatal Nurses.

Simpson KR, Poole JH: *Cervical ripening and induction and augmentation of labor,* Washington, DC, 1998, Association of Women's Health, Obstetric and Neonatal Nurses.

Sprague A, Trepanier MJ: Charting in record time, *AWHONN Lifelines* 3(5):25-30, 1999.

Index

t Indicates table, *italics* indicate
illustration.